Key Concepts in
Palliative
Care

The SAGE Key Concepts series provides students with accessible and authoritative knowledge of the essential topics in a variety of disciplines. Cross-referenced throughout, the format encourages critical evaluation through understanding. Written by experienced and respected academics, the books are indispensable study aids and guides to comprehension.

MOYRA A. BALDWIN AND JAN WOODHOUSE

Key Concepts in
Palliative
Care

First published 2011

SAGE Publications Ltd
1 Oliver's Yard
55 City Road
London EC1Y 1SP

SAGE Publications Inc.
2455 Teller Road
Thousand Oaks, California 91320

SAGE Publications India Pvt Ltd
B 1/I 1 Mohan Cooperative Industrial Area
Mathura Road
New Delhi 110 044

SAGE Publications Asia-Pacific Pte Ltd
33 Pekin Street #02-01
Far East Square
Singapore 048763

Library of Congress Control Number: 2010925117

British Library Cataloguing in Publication data

A catalogue record for this book is available from the British Library

ISBN 978-1-84860-871-9
ISBN 978-1-84860-872-6 (pbk)

Typeset by C&M Digitals (P) Ltd, Chennai, India
Printed by CPI Antony Rowe, Chippenham, Wiltshire
Printed on paper from sustainable resources

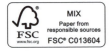

contents

contents

v

contents

vii

key concepts in
palliative care

list of figures

list of tables

key concepts in
palliative care

x

about the editors and contributors

EDITORS

Moyra A. Baldwin, BSc (Hons), MMed Sci. (Clinical Nursing), RN (Adult), SRN, RCNT, RNT, Dip N (London), Cert Ed, Dip Adv Nursing Studies is Senior Lecturer and Programme Leader of the Post Graduate Certificate in Health and Social Care Commissioning, Faculty of Health and Social Care, University of Chester.

Jan Woodhouse, MEd, BN(Hons) Dip N, PGDE, RGN, OND, FETC is Senior Lecturer, Department of Professional Development in Health Care, in the Faculty of Health and Social Care, University of Chester.

CONTRIBUTORS

Julie Bailey-McHale, MSc, BA (Hons), PG Dip Ed, RMN is Senior Lecturer in Mental Health, Isle of Man Department of Health and Social Security (DHSS).

Barbara Beard, MA(Medical Ethics), BA, RGN, RNT, RCNT, ENB 931, Cert Counselling(AEB) is Course Leader, MSc Supportive and Palliative Care at Sheffield Hallam University.

Catherine Black, MA Ed, BA (Hons) Nursing, RN, RNT, Dip in Health Services Management is Senior Lecturer, Isle of Man Department of Health and Social Security (DHSS).

Adrian Bunnell, MSc (Advance Practice), BSc Occupational Therapy is Clinical Specialist Occupational Therapist in the Palliative Care Community Therapy Team, Western Cheshire Primary Care Trust at the Hospice of the Good Shepherd, Chester.

Dorothy Carter is Chair of FOCUS – Forum of Carers and Users of Services – she is also a former carer and former manager at Age Concern, Warrington.

John Costello, RN, PhD is Senior Lecturer in palliative care nursing, School of Nursing, Midwifery and Social Work, University of Manchester.

Sonya Currey, RN (Adult), Dip HE Nursing Studies, BSc (Hons) Specialist Practitioner District Nursing is a District Nurse Sister, Warrington Community Service Unit.

Andrea Dean, Dip HE Nursing Studies, BSc (Hons) Professional Practice (Nursing) is a Research Nurse at Roy Castle Liverpool Lung Project, University of Liverpool Cancer Research Centre.

The Reverend Ian M. Delinger, BSc, BTh (Cantab) is Assistant Chaplain, University of Chester.

John Ellershaw is Professor of Palliative Medicine and Director of Marie Curie Palliative Care Institute at the University of Liverpool.

Shirley Firth, BA (Hons), PG Cert Social Work for Developing Countries, LSE, MA, PhD, SOAS, is a retired writer, lecturer and workshop facilitator. Oxfam, Florissant College, St. Louis, USA; Open University; Universities of Southern Maine (USA), Surrey, Reading, Winchester (King Alfred's College), Southampton.

Yvonne Flood, RGN, RSCN, BSc Children's Community Nursing, PGCE HE, is Lecturer in the School of Nursing and Midwifery at Keele University.

Janice Foster, SRN, DPSN, BSc Hons, RMA is Inpatient Unit Manager, St Ann's Hospice, Manchester.

Helen Fruin, BA (Hons), CQSW, Dip Soc, Admin, PGCE is Senior Lecturer in Practice Learning, Faculty of Health and Social Care, University of Chester.

Joanne Greenwood, MSc, PGCE, BSc (Hons), DipHE (Dist), RGN is Senior Lecturer, Faculty of Health and Social Care, University of Chester.

Richard Griffith, LLM BN DipN, PgdL, RMN, RNT, Cert Ed is Lecturer in Health Law, School of Health Science, Swansea University.

Peter Hartland is Chief Executive of St Luke's Hospice, Sheffield.

Amanda Humphreys, RGN (Adult), Cert Prof Practice, RGN (Childrens), Cert HE, Dip Prof Practice, BSc (Hons), Lecturer / Practice Educator, MA is Team Leader at Hope House Children's Hospice in Shropshire.

Claire Jones, MSc Advanced Practice, Diploma in Physiotherapy is Clinical Specialist Physiotherapist in the Palliative Care Community Therapy Team, Western Cheshire Primary Care Trust and at the Hospice of the Good Shepherd, Chester.

Steve Kirk, SRN, RMN, RNMH, DipHE Palliative Care, MBA was formerly the Chief Executive of St Luke's Hospice, Sheffield.

Dr Richard J. Latten, MB ChB, MRCP (UK) is Clinical Fellow in Palliative Medicine at the Marie Curie Palliative Care Institute, University of Liverpool.

Mzwandile A. Mabhala, FRIPH, MSc (PH), BSc (Hons), PG Cert Ed is Senior Lecturer in Public Health and Epidemiology, Faculty of Health and Social Care, University of Chester.

Karen Manford-Walley, **MEd, BSc(Hons), SCPHN Occupational Health, BSc (Hons), DipHE, RGN, Onc Cert, FP Cert, Gradi OSH, FHEA** is a Senior Lecturer, University of Chester and Oncology Lecturer, Clatterbridge Centre for Oncology, Wirral.

Elizabeth Mason-Whitehead, PhD, BA(Hons), PGDE, SRN, SCM, RHV, ONC is Professor of Social and Health Care at the Faculty of Health and Social Care, University of Chester.

Jill McCarthy, EdD, MSc, BEd (Hons), RGN, SPQ (DN), RNT is Senior Lecturer, Faculty of Health and Social Care, The University of Chester.

Deborah Murphy is National Lead Nurse LCP, Associate Director, Marie Curie Palliative Care Institute, University of Liverpool.

Stephanie Neill, MSc Accounting and Finance, Diploma in Management Studies (DMS), Certified Diploma Accounting and Finance (C.Dip AF), HNC Business Studies, is Treasurer and service user at FOCUS.

Sue Padmore, Med, BA (Hons) RM, RN, Diploma in Holistic Therapies (IIHHT) is Senior Lecturer, Faculty of Health and Social Care, University of Chester.

Joy Parkes, MSc Clinical Skills In Practice; BSc (Hons) Nursing Studies; RNT; RN; RM; IIHHT Dip in Health and Holistic Therapies, is Senior Lecturer Adult Nursing and Practice Lead at the Faculty of Health and Social Care at the University of Chester.

Natalie Pattison, RN, BSc (Hons), MSc, Cancer (Adult) Diploma is Clinical Nursing Research Fellow at the Royal Marsden Hospital, Surrey.

Sheila Payne, BA (Hons), RN, Dip N, PhD, C Psychol is Help the Hospices Chair in Hospice Studies, International Observatory on End of Life Care, Division of Health Research at Lancaster University.

Sue Phillips, RGN, RHV, BA (Hons) Nursing Education, MSc is Senior Lecturer, Faculty of Health and Social Care, University of Chester.

Lynda Prescott, MA, BA (Hons), RNT, RN is Nurse Educator and Team Leader, Sydney West Area Health Service in New South Wales, Australia.

Jane Quigley, MSc, PGDE, RGN, DN, Nurse Prescribing is Senior Lecturer, Faculty of Health and Social Care, University of Chester.

Sue Read, PhD, MA, RNMH, Cert Ed (FE), Cert Bereavement Studies is Reader in Learning Disability Nursing at Keele University.

Victoria Ridgway, RN, BSc (Hons), MA Gerontology, PGDE is Programme Leader/Senior Lecturer, Faculty of Health and Social Care, University of Chester.

Pat Rose, MSc, BSc (Hons), Dip N, PG Cert Ed, RHV, RN (Child), RN (Adult) Honorary Research Fellow, Faculty of Health and Social Care, University of Chester.

Dion Smyth, RGN, PG Dip, Cert Ed, ONC is Lecturer-Practitioner in cancer and palliative care at Birmingham City University.

Virginia C. Williams, MSc PG Cert Palliative Care, BSc (Hons) Specialist Practitioner, RN, Dip HE (Nursing) is Clinical Nurse Specialist Palliative Care (Macmillan) for Liverpool Primary Care Trust, Edge Hill Health Centre in Liverpool.

Debbie Wyatt, MSc, BA (Hons), DPSN, Cert Ed, RNT, RGN, ENB 237 is Senior Lecturer at Faculty of Health and Social Care, University of Chester and Macmillan Lecturer at Clatterbridge Centre for Oncology, Wirral.

preface

The concept of palliative care has grown over the last half-century, from local provision at dedicated hospices looking after patients with cancer, to a global awareness that considers all the measures needed at the end of life, irrespective of the diagnosis. Subsequently the knowledge base of palliative care has expanded exponentially. It has moved from the minimum of giving effective pain relief by medical staff to embrace a wide range of approaches by all members of the multidisciplinary team, and others, who care for the patient and their carers. It has also moved from just being an end-of-life service to one that is considered from the moment of diagnosis to the subsequent bereavement period of the carers. A glance down the list of key concepts on the contents page will give testament to the diversity of knowledge that palliative care encompasses.

One of those concepts is that of research and today there is much emphasis placed on evidence-based practices, whatever discipline you happen to be working in. Yet palliative care cannot always be guided by the gold standard of research, randomised controlled trials, because of the ethical implications and time-bound aspects of such methods. Hence evidence in palliative care is often gathered by 'what works for the patient, not other patients but this patient'. Hence there is a patient-centred approach that naturally emerges. The use of the Internet has enabled a global sharing of what works and what doesn't and this allows a further growth of knowledge. It also gives weight to opinion-based arguments, where the palliative care expert is drawing on known case studies and observations. As such, this flies in the face of the concept of evidence-based practices but palliative care teams are pragmatic and will try most things if it brings a benefit to the patient. Hence those readers expecting to find treatment protocols in the concepts of symptom management chapters are going to be disappointed, instead they are encouraged to view the patient holistically – to consider all the elements that impact on the patient socially, physically, psychologically and spiritually.

When this is done palliative care practitioners will probably realize that there is a limit to their knowledge and that there is a need to involve others in the multidisciplinary team. Therefore the concepts in this book are drawn from a variety of professions and levels within those professions, which hopefully demonstrates that there has been a team effort in the formulation of the content.

One concept that may seem to be missing is that of physician-assisted suicide and euthanasia, although it is touched upon within a few of the chapters, and that is because this is a book aimed at the practitioner, predominately in the United Kingdom, where the topic is frequently debated but is not enshrined in law. If or when such legislation is passed then it will need to be included as a topic in its own right. Until then the practitioner should be aware of the debates that are going on around this highly emotive topic for sooner or later you can be sure that a patient, or their relative, is going to raise it when faced with a life-limiting diagnosis.

The concepts contained within this book aim to 'give a little about a lot' rather than 'a lot about a little', they are an overview of the elements of palliative care and we hope that the reader finds plenty to stimulate thought, to compare aspects to practice, and to debate with others.

Moyra A. Baldwin and Jan Woodhouse

key concepts in
palliative care

acknowledgements

We wish to thank our palliative care colleagues who have contributed to this book and have been willing to pass on their expertise and knowledge to others.

Special thanks go to Barbara Holliday, whose quiet patience and diligence in all things administrative have helped in the completion of this book.

We would also like to thank our colleagues in the Faculty of Health and Social Care, University of Chester, as well as those at Sage – Emma Paterson, Alison Poyner and Zoë Elliott-Fawcett for their ongoing encouragement, support and guidance.

acknowledgements

xvii

introduction

MOYRA A. BALDWIN AND JAN WOODHOUSE

'There's glory for you!'
'I don't know what you mean by glory,' Alice said.
'I meant, "there's a nice-knock down argument for you!"'
'But "glory" doesn't mean "a nice-knock down argument", Alice objected.
'When I use a word,' Humpty Dumpty said in a rather scornful tone, 'it means just what I choose it to mean – neither more nor less.'

(Lewis Carroll, 1832–1989)

Investment in the organisation and management of palliative care, over recent years, has resulted in a broadening access to palliative care services. Cognizance of common, and often complex, concepts that influence and impact on patients' lives, as well as on the lives of carers, will enable integration of the essence of palliative care into practice in primary, secondary and tertiary health care environments.

By their nature, concepts are abstract representations of reality, this book examines the key concepts of palliative care, applying our understanding of each concept through practice examples. The number and title of chapters, devised as a result of a surveying students', palliative care practitioners', and educators' opinions of the concepts, pertinent to their practice experience, are intended to give the reader a broad and comprehensive perspective of the concepts that are relevant and significant to palliative care.

The book is aimed at a variety of practitioners working both within and outwith the speciality of palliative care. The readership includes all health and social care professionals who will be able to use the book as a reference point or supplementary reading, reading one concept at a time as an introduction to an essential aspect of palliative care.

Fifty concepts are organised in alphabetical order, for ease of reference and chapters, with the exception of Chapter 33, arranged as follows. First, the concept is defined within a broad parameter and within the context of palliative care. Next, key points associated with the concept are listed, providing an outline of the chapter, and are subsequently developed in the discussion section. A concluding, practical application of the concept illustrates its relevance to palliative care practice. Finally, readers are guided to extend their palliative care knowledge with reference to related concepts and further literature. Chapter 33 is written by a service user and a carer and includes four case studies clearly illustrating clients' perspective.

The authors have been chosen for their expertise and experience. This gives a wide range of authorship, from carers to palliative care consultants, from general nurses to Macmillan nurses, and from educators to policy-makers.

Hence, a gamut of inter-professionals gives weight to the individual concepts, which befits the palliative care philosophy.

Developing understanding of concepts comes from their use in practice and, rather than Humpty Dumpty's idiosyncratic notion in the story of *Through the Looking Glass*, we trust that we have examined concepts as Alice does and illuminated the key concepts of palliative care by providing readers with a concise understanding of each.

1 agencies: resources for adults with a palliative care need in the UK

Helen Fruin

DEFINITION

An adult requiring palliative care can be defined as someone 'whose disease is not responsive to curative treatment' (World Health Organisation, 1990, cited in Gehlert and Browne, 2006), and who will, or currently does, require 'end of life care' (Department of Health, 2006). The range of agencies specifically organised and available for patients, service users and their carers is extensive. The adult age range, incorporating people across younger, middle, and primarily older ages, together with differentials of location, disease, prognosis, gender, race, culture, religion, affluence, and so on, gives some indication that the agencies required to encompass both the specific and general needs of patients with palliative care requirements need to be vast in range and widely available. Rather than define or list the possible resources that might be required for patients and their families, a broad categorizing of the UK sectors that palliative care agencies may be attributed to with examples of the types of agencies that exist are explored below. 'Local variations' will, however, 'grossly distort equity and efficiency in individual areas' (Netten and Beecham, 1993). Also, many agencies contacted by individuals may be 'generalist rather than specialist' (Roe and Beech, 2005), such as nursing homes, which illustrates the extent and scope of resources available for adults with a palliative care need in the UK.

KEY POINTS

- Three main sectors encompass the majority of agencies concerned with palliative care. These are:
  o voluntary sector,
  o private sector,
  o statutory sector.

- Some may be jointly funded or managed within or across these sectors.
- Accessibility and suitability of agencies need to be determined to offer the best value and use of resources for individuals and families or carers.

DISCUSSION

Voluntary sector agencies

Many of the voluntary agencies are registered as charities. Financial support is crucial to the survival of these organisations and, in some cases particularly for the smaller charities, funding can be precarious to such an extent that service users may be asked, or feel obliged, to offer a donation. Most hospices operate as charities; '80% of hospices are independent of the NHS', with only '34% of their funding from government' (Peckham and Meerabeau, 2007). National agencies stemming from the hospice movement include Marie Curie hospices, day care and outreach services, Macmillan nurse advice and support at home, and agencies that provide advice on specific medical conditions (which may or may not be of a palliative nature) via leaflets, telephone or websites, such as the British Heart Foundation, and others concerned with various types of cancers.

Voluntary agencies that are accessed by people affected by conditions which may become terminal include generalist organisations such as Age Concern or religious-based agencies which can offer either, or both, practical and spiritual support, for example, Nugent Care Society and other Roman Catholic-based care agencies. Carers, also, often draw support from these agencies and will utilize others specifically designed for them such as Crossroads. Crossroads provides, among other support, a domiciliary sitting service to allow carers a short break. For many patients who have palliative care needs, there are issues other than managing pain or unpleasant symptoms and these can be almost as distressing as the terminal condition itself, for example, unresolved family relationships and the care of surviving partners and children: significant support can be obtained from counselling agencies such as the Salvation Army's Family Tracing Service. Often overlooked but of crucial concern for their distressed owners is the care of pets. There are animal welfare agencies such as the Cinnamon Trust which aims to keep owners with their pets for as long as possible and arranges for their future care (Cooke, 2000).

Private sector agencies

Agencies within the private sector may be funded entirely by service users or receive some funding from other sectors, for example, statutory agencies. Most are profit-making concerns though profits will vary from barely covering costs to those making more substantial returns: location and cost to service users will determine the accessibility of these services. Agencies within the private sector include residential and nursing homes (some may be condition-specific, most are generalist), clinics and hospitals, and domiciliary care/nursing agencies providing brief visits or longer shifts in the final stages of an illness. Some private sector agencies are national organisations, for example, BUPA-managed homes, others are individual to their own locations.

Statutory sector agencies

The statutory sector provides the bulk of primary health and social care for patients and service users with the UK NHS being the main direct provider, or indirect commissioner, of funding and services. As with the voluntary and private agencies, the statutory sector offers a lengthy list of possible services, and again, these may be specific or general to the condition or needs of a patient requiring palliative care. Typical services from pre- to actual diagnosis and progression include those of general practitioners, district nurses, clinics, wards, pharmacies and therapies, for example, treatment therapies such as chemotherapy and 'activity' therapies such as occupational and physiotherapies. As with the complexity of people's social conditions in relation to their palliative condition, medical staff often need to address multi-health needs where other issues, such as a heart condition, may complicate the treatment and management of a patient, and thus require input from other specialist agencies.

Care assessment and management of agency input

From a social care/social work perspective, resources may be jointly funded or managed with, or by, health staff. To ensure service users receive optimal palliative care, statutory agency representatives, for example, nurses or social workers, assessing the needs of the person are best equipped if they are knowledgeable about a range of agencies that may 'best fit' the current, and changing needs of the service user. Only a few years ago it was observed (Department of Health, 2006) that '50% of people ... would like to be cared for and die at home if … terminally ill, (but) …' at that time only 20% died at home. Assessors, whether from health care or social care sectors, will assess individuals and families according to their discipline and expertise, refer to relevant agencies where appropriate, and aim to offer as inclusively as possible information and guidance about the services *realistically* available and suitable for the person's needs.

In social work/care, the drive towards self-directed or personalised care whereby individuals and their family may be given resources to research, recruit and manage their own care services at home will, probably, encourage the growth of voluntary and private sector agencies to support such care packages. This will genuinely enable a more personalised service for people with palliative care needs *if* a sufficient 'mixed economy' (Peckham and Meerabeau, 2007) of all the sectors, as well as the most important element of family and friends' input, is readily accessible at the point of need. Issues of sensitive and accurate assessments, information sharing, criteria for funding and resource allocation, timing, and the overall management of the range of agencies involved need to be carefully administered to avoid the criticism of 'quantity, but not necessarily quality' (Parker, 2005) for service users, and to make the process of palliative care as positive and supportive as possible.

Quality of care

Agencies, like individuals, vary in the quality of care they deliver. While agencies can be expected to adhere to their own and government standards, the governance of quality also comes from the 'customer' via service users' and carers' feedback, as well as the commissioning agency such as Social Services departments. Nevertheless, it is apparent that there are gaps in assessing agency quality which, perhaps, is not surprising given the vast range requiring regular inspection and collation of feedback. Problems may arise where vulnerable individuals are too ill, frightened or distracted to complain about, or criticise, the services received. This also applies to their families and friends, regardless of whether agencies are residential, domiciliary or clinical. Consistent and objective use of agencies, along with appropriately channelled feedback about the quality of the services they provide (perhaps through star ratings), can provide individuals and assessors with knowledge and power to make informed choices to engage or continue with selected agencies.

agencies

5

PRACTICAL APPLICATION OF THE CONCEPT

Kay is 72 years of age, and her cancer is now advanced. Kay has already referred herself (and her family have) to some agencies, for example, her local GP and social services. She has had a range of NHS interventions which professionals have arranged, with her consent, including diagnostic tests, consultations, surgery, therapies, prescriptions, equipment/aids.

Kay's social worker from an older persons team has assessed her and her carer, her husband Jim, to discuss care options. This is also done, ideally, in partnership with a medical colleague, GP or nurse. Discussions on hospices, nursing homes and domiciliary care/nursing are on-going, as well as other details such as applying for Attendance Allowance (the local Welfare Rights or Citizen's Advice Bureau is recommended). Jim's support is also assessed and discussed, and he would welcome the idea of a volunteer from his local church or Crossroads to come in, just once a week for now, to allow him to go out for a couple of hours. His health and stress will also need to be monitored and supported as well as Kay's if he is to support her through to the end.

Kay, Jim and their family have already been on websites and telephoned help-lines to research her condition and possible agencies that might help. However, they still need advice as to what is available locally, what eligibility criteria are applied, how long any waiting list might be, whether there are any costs, and crucially, whether they will be professional, reliable and caring. The social worker and her health colleague, from their experience, continue to give as much objective information as they can to help Kay and Jim choose the most appropriate agencies and options, as both their needs will change through Kay's illness.

See also: finance issues; multi-disciplinary teams; patient choices and preferences; policy drivers; resources and caring for the carers

FURTHER READING

Cooke, H. (2000) *When Someone Dies: A Practical Guide to Holistic Care at the End of Life*. Oxford: Reed Educational and Professional Publishing Ltd.

Peckham, S. and Meerabeau, L. (2007) *Social Policy for Nurses and the Helping Professions*, 2nd edn. Maidenhead: Open University Press.

REFERENCES

Cooke, H. (2000) *When Someone Dies: A Practical Guide to Holistic Care at the End of Life*. Oxford: Reed Educational and Professional Publishing Ltd.

Department of Health (2006) *Our Health, Our Care, Our Say: A New Direction for Community Service*. London: Department of Health.

Gehlert, S. and Browne, T. (2006) *Handbook of Health Social Work*. Chichester: John Wiley & Sons, Inc.

Netten, A. and Beecham, J. (1993) *Costing Community Care*. Cambridge: Cambridge University Press.

Parker, J. (ed.) (2005) *Aspects of Social work and Palliative Care*. London: Quay Books.

Peckham, S. and Meerabeau, L. (2007) *Social Policy for Nurses and the Helping Professions*, 2nd edn. Maidenhead: Open University Press.

Roe, B. and Beech, R. (2005) *Intermediate and Continuing Care*. London: Blackwell Publishing.

2 attributes of palliative caring

Moyra A. Baldwin

DEFINITION

In her exploration of the concept of caring Rose (2008) notes that caring cannot be defined neatly in a succinct statement. It can be described as a concept that encompasses behaviours and attitudes that healthcare professionals engage in to help another, such as a patient. Helping is achieved through the relationship between two people: the carer and the cared for. Similarly, in palliative care, a characteristic of caring is the relationship between the healthcare professional and the person with a palliative care need and, or, a member of family, friend or a healthcare professional colleague. The importance of this helping relationship is apparent in the philosophies, guidance and mission statements published by the World Health Organisation, Department of Health and local hospices respectively, and so it appears that there is international, national and local implied understanding of palliative caring. This helping relationship within the confines of palliative care will be examined to provide the focus for discussing the attributes of palliative caring in this chapter.

KEY POINTS

- Palliative caring involves holistic care.
- Attributes of palliative care include developing therapeutic relationship between the carer and cared-for, as well as professional colleagues.
- Therapeutic relationships require that the carer individualises care for the person with end-of-life needs as well as the individual's family.
- Palliative caring attributes are encompassed in companionship, compassion and competence.

DISCUSSION

When concepts such as palliative caring are, inherently, understood by the people involved in the work yet not necessarily clearly defined, a concept analysis can help provide shared meaning. In the international arena Meghani (2004) conducted a concept analysis of palliative care and showed that, for an American audience, palliative care has four components. First, it involves total, active and individualized patient care, second, it includes family support, third, interdisciplinary teamwork, and finally effective communication. What Meghani identifies is the therapeutic, helping relationship that is essential in caring for individuals and families in the palliative stage of the person's illness. Others also identify the significance of the therapeutic relationship (see Table 2.1), for example, Degner et al. (1991) and Canning et al. (2007).

Canning et al. (2007), in their investigation into the domains of Specialist Palliative Care Nursing Practice, explicitly noted that therapeutic relationships were fundamental and connected the remaining areas of palliative care for the specialist practitioners. The other domains of specialist palliative nursing noted by these researchers were complex supportive care, collaborative practice, leadership and improving practice, all of which can be interpreted as components of helping relationships. In less explicit terms but nevertheless by inference, Degner's et al. (1991), seven critical nursing behaviours (listed in Table 2.1) in care of the dying similarly acknowledge the value of the therapeutic relationship in palliative caring. Degner et al. interviewed 10 educators and 10 nurse practitioners and found that caring behaviours associated with care of the dying from a Canadian perspective included what I will label reactive and proactive interventions. The study identified both positive and negative qualities in the seven behaviours which suggests that the attributes of palliative caring demand the ability, first, to recognize the need for, followed by the use of, a repertoire of effective caring attributes. One can conclude from this that self-awareness of personal knowledge is also an important attribute of palliative caring.

Holism and holistic care

Holism and holistic care are associated with much of the literature on palliative care and appear to combine the bio-psycho-social aspects of the person. Some assert that holism and, subsequently, holistic care, are concerned with more than this. Holism captures the values of compassion, respect, open-mindedness competence, and self-caring according the British Holistic Medical Association (BHMA) (undated). This is portrayed in studies that explore the encounters and meaning healthcare professionals ascribe to their roles in palliative caring. Dunniece and Slevin's (2002) study of the lived experiences of seven accomplished nurses who had worked for a minimum of two years in a range of palliative care settings reveals a pattern of holistic, individualised care, which is both proactive and reactive, and demonstrates the importance of self-awareness, as identified by the BHMA. Additionally, companionship is an important attribute for the participants in Dunniece and Slevin's (2002) study. The participants described companionship in what they explained as 'being with'. The notion of 'being with' involves an encounter with patients, at the end of life, in which both holism and individuality are combined.

Total, active individualised patient care and family support

In the International Observatory on End of Life Care publication of professionals' accounts of their caring experiences, the cared-for individual is no

Table 2.1 Attributes of palliative caring

WHO (2010)	NICE (2004)	Meghani (2004)	Davies and Oberle (1990)	Canning et al. (2007)	Degner et al. (1991)	Thomas (2003) GSF	Dunniece and Slevin (2002)	Barnard et al. (2006)
Improves the quality of life	Best quality of life	Total active and individualized patient care	Valuing	Complex supportive care	Responding during the death scene	Patient centred	Knowing the bigger picture	Doing everything you can
Prevention and relief of suffering	Pain and symptom relief	Family support	Connecting	Collaborative practice	Providing comfort	Patient and carer empowerment – to be active members of the team	Time: movement and measure	Developing closeness
Integrates psychological and spiritual care	Support to patient and family	Interdisciplinary teamwork	Doing for	Leadership	Responding to anger	Security, comfort and support for patients and carers at home	Ethical dimensions	Working as a team
Pain and symptom relief		Effective communication	Finding meaning	Improving practice	Enhancing personal growth	Staff confidence, communication and co-working	Knowing and 'minding yourself'	Maintaining myself
Support to patient and family			Empowering	Therapeutic relationship	Responding to colleagues		The 'just' and 'simply' of practice	
			Preserving integrity		Enhancing the quality of life during dying		The embodiment of 'being with'	
					Responding to the family		Unseen tutors	

longer perceived by professionals as an object of care (McDermott, 2009). Over a period of 30 years healthcare professionals, mainly doctors and nurses, acknowledge that the person, with a cancer diagnosis being cared for at the end of life, is an autonomous, self-governing person. Despite the author's (McDermott) caution about professionals' lack of a clear understanding of autonomy, the study shows that palliative caring encompasses the concept of individualised patient care.

In a specific and local setting personalised care is, again, explicit in the framework for community palliative care. The Gold Standards Framework (GSF) (Thomas, 2003), the UK's model of good practice for community palliative care aspires to provide total, active and individualised patient care for patients nearing the end of life by using the seven key standards: communication, co-ordination, control of symptoms, continuity of care, continued learning, carer support, and care in the dying phase. In that the therapeutic relationship is key to palliative caring, it requires that the healthcare practitioner personalises care for individuals and, indeed, their families. From the discussion above it can be seen that palliative caring focuses on a patient's and family's needs, and demands professional responsiveness. Davies and Oberle's (1990) model, a qualitative study, identifying the dimensions of the supportive role of the nurse in palliative care typifies the components of holism, holistic care, total active individualized patient care and family support. Particular aspects of the model that apply here are the valuing, connecting, empowering and doing for dimensions. Below the model can be seen to fit the teamworking and communication.

Teamwork and effective communication

Meghani (2004) and Barnard et al.'s (2006) studies clearly identify the importance of teamwork in palliative caring. Speck (2006), on the other hand, offers a contrary view of the effectiveness, or necessity, of palliative care teamwork. From the patients' perspectives, it appears that teamwork is not how they view palliative care. Nevertheless, the team has an important function, not only securing patients' needs but also sustaining the professional palliative carer (see Barnard et al., 2006 and first issue of *End of Life Care* journal (Payne, 2007), for further details). Other studies imply teamwork as an attribute (see Table 2.1). In addition to studies that show teamwork's importance to individual professions, NICE (2004: 7, recommendation 3) recommended that teams should implement processes that would ensure effective communication, both within and between teams. The variety of teams from health and social care agencies and service providers with whom patients have contact requires the mechanisms to which NICE refers in order to secure continuity of care. This appears to exist, according to Payne (2007), who describes effective team working relationships whereby collaboration between a range of healthcare professionals and social workers, to develop packages of care or discharge arrangements, enables palliative caring. Collaboration between and within professionals and agencies thus allows holistic approaches to ensure individualised care and, of course, teamwork.

From the discussion above drawing on evidence from research, national and local directives, it can be seen that palliative caring involves individual, holistic care.

This is achieved by developing therapeutic relationship between the carer and cared-for, including the family and professional colleagues. Being able to 'break the connection' and secure one's own 'integrity' are important as the professionals also face elements of loss, grief and bereavement in their encounters with patients and families. These attributes of palliative caring are explicitly expressed in the literature, for example, Davies and Oberle (1990) and Barnard et al. (2006). In summary, the attributes of palliative caring are companionship, compassion and competence and these can be seen to be present in Ruth's care below.

PRACTICAL APPLICATION OF THE CONCEPT

Ruth, a 58-year-old lady admitted to the hospice with symptoms of nausea and vomiting as a result of an advanced mediastinal cancer and superior vena cava obstruction (SVCO). Ruth is nearing the end stage of her life and plans are being made for her return home. Amanda, her named nurse, is coordinating the plans with other members of the team at the hospice, social worker and voluntary agencies in order to support Ruth at home. A day before her discharge Ruth became breathless, was nauseated and had three episodes of vomiting. Amanda thought that Ruth's condition was due to her deteriorating SVCO and discussed this with her colleagues. After a number of discussions between the palliative care team and the local cancer centre, it was clear that there was a strong possibility that Ruth might not manage to get home. Amanda spoke with Ruth and, with her permission, spoke with her close family too. Both Amanda and the hospice doctor spoke with Ruth and found out the interpretation she made of her symptoms. Between them they showed competence, compassion and companionship. They used their knowledge of symptoms and recognised worsening symptoms. They collaborated with the wider members of the team at the cancer centre and, having realised that Ruth was dying, communicated openly and compassionately with her. The compassion and companionship shown to Ruth enabled her to let the team know that she was aware that her condition was more advanced than she had hoped. Plans continued toward managing an afternoon visit home.

See also: *communication; multi-disciplinary teamwork*

FURTHER READING

Payne, S., Seymour, J., and Ingleton, C. (eds) (2008) *Palliative Care Nursing: Principles and Evidence for Practice*, 2nd edn. Maidenhead: Open University Press.
Speck, P. (ed.) (2006) *Teamwork in Palliative Care: Fulfilling or Frustrating?* Oxford: Oxford University Press.

REFERENCES

Barnard, A., Hollingum, C. and Hartfield, B. (2006) 'Going on a journey: understanding palliative care nursing', *International Journal of Palliative Nursing*, 12(1): 6–12.
British Holistic Medical Association (BHMA) website. www.bhma.org/modules.php?op=modload&name=PagEd&file=index&topic_id=0&page_id=50 accessed 12 March 2009.

attributes

11

Canning, D., Rosenberg, J.P. and Yates, P. (2007) 'Therapeutic relationships in specialist palliative care nursing practice', *International Journal of Palliative Nursing*, 13(5): 222–9.

Centre for Palliative Care Research and Education (CPCRE) (2007) 'Competency standards for specialist palliative care practice'. Available at: www.health.qld.gov.au/cpcre/pdf/compstand.pdf accessed 20 September 2009.

Davies, B. and Oberle, K. (1990) 'Dimensions of the supportive role of the nurse in palliative care', *Oncology Nursing Forum*, 17(1): 87–94.

Degner, L.F., Gow, C.M. and Thompson, L.A. (1991) 'Critical nursing behaviours in care for the dying', *Cancer Nursing*, 14(5): 246–53.

Dunniece, U. and Slevin, E. (2002) 'Giving voice to the less articulated knowledge of palliative nursing: an interpretative study', *International Journal of Palliative Nursing*, 8(1): 13–20.

Meghani, S.H. (2004) 'A concept analysis of palliative care in the United States', *Journal of Advanced Nursing*, 46(2): 152–61.

McDermott, L. (2009) 'Professional writings on caring for people with cancer at the end of life'. Available at: www.eolc-observatory.net/patientcarer/professional_literature.htm accessed 12 March 2009.

National Institute for Clinical Excellence (2004) *Guidance on Cancer Services Improving Supportive and Palliative Care for Adults with Cancer: The Manual*. London: NICE.

Payne, M. (2007) 'Know your colleagues: role of social work in end-of-life care', *End of Life Care*, 1(1): 69–73.

Rose, P. (2008) 'Caring', in E. Mason-Whitehead, A. McIntosh, A. Bryan and T. Mason (eds), *Key Concepts in Nursing*. London: Sage, pp. 42–8.

Speck, P. (ed.) (2006) *Teamwork in Palliative Care: Fulfilling or Frustrating?* Oxford: Oxford University Press.

Thomas, K. (2003) *Caring for the Dying at Home*. Abingdon: Radcliffe Medical Press.

WHO (2010) *WHO Definition of Palliative Care*. Available at: www.who.int/cancer/palliative/definition/en accessed 4 September 2010.

3 caring for the adult: 'a reversal of roles'

Virginia C. Williams

DEFINITION

This chapter will focus on the roles and responsibilities we encounter when caring for adults. Definitions of the terms used will be considered and it will also reflect on how these roles are influenced when the adult's condition becomes palliative. Morris and Thomas (2001) indicate that the term 'carer' is relatively recent and is used generally in health research to cover a range of situations which usually involve irreversible impairment in a cared-for person and concomitant provision of help with activities of daily living. There does not appear to be a clear definition of what defines an 'adult' although traditionally these are years that are viewed as one long plateau that separates childhood from old age (Boyle, 2008). Others choose to place the population into boxes defined by age brackets, for example, 60+ are often described as older adults. It makes no sense to categorise in this manner as there are some adults aged 80+ who live very active and varied lives and others whose lives are restricted. It needs to be remembered that there is nothing predictable about the lives of people who have attained a certain age (Bailey, 2002) and there is little rationale for categorising adults beyond the need to achieve a form of orderliness in healthcare statistics or society at large. Clearly stereotyping anyone over a certain age reflects the kind of society we live in.

KEY POINTS

- A culture of caring for adults.
- Differences between the family, lay carer and the professional.
- The impact of palliative diagnosis on family life.
- Role reversal for carers.

DISCUSSION

A culture of caring

Historically, the older generation has lived in an environment where there was initially no health service free at the point of delivery. Instead, there was the support of a family, whose duty was to care and where women were at home managing with whatever resources they had available (Cook, 2005). Caregiving is embedded in a range of social relationships with family, friends and neighbours, which reflect various caring roles and responsibilities. When disability or illness strikes one or other in a relationship, the experiences of the carer can reflect the gender role expectations of society. A woman's caring role may become an extension of her role as a wife, and this can be taken for granted by all concerned (McClure, 2001). Indeed, Khalili (2007) purports that the role and responsibility of the caregiver are often increased to not only maintaining the care of the patient, but also to sustain prior roles and responsibilities within the household. This is in addition to continuing to work full-time or part-time, as women have now become an established part of the workforce, adopting family life around a full-time or part-time career (Cook, 2005).

Family lay carer or professional?

Pickard and Glendinning (2002) indicate that there are several factors which distinguish family care givers from professionals. It is suggested that family care givers believe that their role forms part of a familial relationship comprising of love and duty. Importantly, it is limitless, not contained within a specific time-frame, and characterised by spontaneity when unexpected events or crises occur. In addition to this, family carers develop a differing expertise to professional staff, in that they have an understanding of the individual and become adept at focusing on specific tasks, as opposed to the professional, who focuses on the whole person. There are characteristics that set professionals apart from family care-givers, including professional detachment and the experience of working within a time-limited and bounded routine. The activities of professional staff are circumscribed by the time limits imposed by other requirements of their caseload. In contrast, lay-carers' contributions can be open-ended, which in turn, due to the time spent, can allow the carer to build up person-centred expertise.

Impact of palliative diagnosis

The impact of a life-limiting diagnosis, such as cancer, is a deep and life-changing experience and the effect of this disease on the family and friends of somebody with such a diagnosis can be intense. Indeed, life may change quite fundamentally as a result of the diagnosis. For example, giving up work or moving closer to the individual with a life-limiting disease in order that appropriate and supportive care may be given. Important aspects of family life may have to be altered, holidays may no longer be planned or financial difficulties may be incurred. The carer may feel that the person whom they knew has been lost and this can be disturbing to the family and is perhaps even harder to recognise or know how to support (Plant, 2002). The carer situation can alter dramatically in the levels of uncertainty of outcome, timescale and physical impairment of the patient. These changes impact not only on the patient with the disease, but also those living with and caring for the patient (Morris and Thomas, 2001). The social impact of the disease and its effect on family relationships become part of the day-to-day living, with the use of protection strategies, such as avoidance and denial, which are both a way of caring and a way of coping with the fear and uncertainty created by the illness.

Role reversal

The role of the informal carer is highly idealised by society, where images are evoked of self-sacrifice, patience and understanding. Over a 30- or 40-year span, there may be a complete reversal in roles, as the once helpless infants grow towards middle age and perhaps eventually take on the care of their aged parents (Frude, 2000). The relationship between parent and child is an important source of security throughout life and any disruption to this can cause difficulties which may manifest themselves psychologically at a later date. Although every child knows that eventually the time will come when they will lose their parent, and the supportive role that has been forged, it is seen as much more acceptable that death occurs due to old age, rather than death from cancer. Difficulties can arise when the child has to step out of the role of being a child into the role of being a parent, caring for somebody who is no longer able to care for themselves. Any situation in which a family member requires care and support can involve a degree of role reversal and it may be suggested that adults can become sandwiched between the layers of caring for their own children and their parents (Wright and Leahey, 2005). They can feel besieged on both sides: teenagers asking for more freedom and grandparents asking for more support; with the growing trend of women to have children later in life and seniors living longer, this double demand for attention, and resources, most likely will intensify.

Current trends within palliative care are leading towards the move away from in-patient care to care in the community, and on average, it is suspected that patients can spend up to 90% of their last year of life at home, being cared for informally with primary health care team back-up. Evidence shows that the majority of patients with palliative care needs would choose to spend the end of their life at home (Morris and Thomas, 2001), although ensuring adequate care provision is in place remains problematic. Caring for adults with a diagnosis such as cancer involves not only dealing with the cancer diagnosis, but the symptoms of the cancer itself, which can be wide and varied. Negotiating the transition from living with cancer, or another life-limiting disease, to palliation can be difficult and opportunities must be seized to provide information and support to family caregivers (Khalili, 2007).

PRACTICAL APPLICATION OF THE CONCEPT

Ida is a 69-year-old woman who is heavily reliant on her daughter Sarah, due to residual effects from a stroke two years previously. Her mobility is limited and she requires some assistance with her daily activities. She refuses to have outside agencies to assist in her daily needs, preferring instead that Sarah takes care of her. This places a burden on Sarah as she works full-time and has two young children. Sarah often feels torn between the commitments to her own children and the expectation that she should be there to care for her mother. Sarah finds it difficult to manage Ida's care needs alongside running the family home, as well as maintaining her full-time job. This, coupled with Ida's reluctance to allow outside assistance and the expectation that Sarah should help her, causes a strain on the relationship.

Ida has recently been experiencing headaches and impaired vision and investigations have discovered that she has a malignant brain tumour. Her prognosis is poor and she makes it clear that she wishes to stay at home at the end of her life, and wants Sarah to care for her. She reluctantly allows the district nurses to deliver some of her nursing care. Despite undergoing intensive treatment, her condition deteriorates rapidly, her needs become greater, and Sarah reduces her working hours temporarily in order to provide end of life care.

See also: caring for the carers; caring for the older person; caring for young people; information technology; patient choices and preferences

FURTHER READING

Department of Health (2001) *National Service Framework for Older People*. London: Department of Health.

Piercy, J. (2002) 'The plight of the informal carer', in R. Charlton (ed.), *Primary Palliative Care: Death, Dying and Bereavement in the Community*. Abingdon: Radcliffe Medical Press, pp. 143–53.

REFERENCES

Bailey, C. (2002) 'The needs of older people', in J. Horner and C. Bailey (eds), *Cancer Nursing, Care in Context*. Oxford: Blackwell Science, pp. 496–507.

Boyle, J. (2008) 'Transcultural perspectives in the nursing care of adults', in M. Andrews and J. Boyle (eds), *Transcultural Concepts in Nursing Care*. Philadelphia: Lippincott Williams & Williams, pp. 146–67.

Cook, L. (2005) 'Demography and social change', in S. Lawton, J. Cantrell and J. Harris (eds), *District Nursing: Providing Care in a Supportive Context*. Edinburgh: Elsevier Churchill Livingston, pp. 35–48.

Frude, N. (2000) 'The family: A psychological perspective', in P. Gastrell and J. Edwards (eds), *Community Health Nursing: Frameworks for Practice*. London: Bailliere Tindall, pp. 92–103.

Khalili, Y. (2007) 'Ongoing transitions: the impact of a malignant brain tumour on patient and family', *Canadian Journal of Neuroscience Nursing*, 28(3): 5–13.

McClure, L. (2001) 'Family caregivers and community nurses: co-experts in care', in V. Hyde (ed.), *Community Nursing and Health Care: Insights and Innovations*. London: Arnold Publishers, pp. 95–118.

Morris, S.M. and Thomas, C. (2001) 'The carers' place in the cancer situation: where does the carer stand in the medical setting?', *European Journal of Palliative Care*, 10: 87–95.

Pickard, S., and Glendinning, C. (2002) 'Comparing and contrasting the role of family carers and nurses in the domestic healthcare of frail older people', *Health and Social Care in the Community*, 10(3): 144–50.

Plant, H. (2002) 'The impact of cancer on the family', in J. Corner and C. Bailey, (eds), *Cancer Nursing: Care in Context*. Oxford: Blackwell Science, pp. 86–99.

Wright, L. and Leahey, M. (2005) *Nurses and Families: A Guide to Family Assessment and Intervention*. Philadelphia: FA Davis Company.

key concepts in palliative care

16

4 caring for the carers

Sheila Payne

DEFINITION

According to the National Institute for Health and Clinical Excellence: 'Carers, who may or may not be family members, are lay people in a close supportive role who share in the illness experience of the patient and who undertake vital care work and emotion management' (NICE, 2004: 155). The same source also defines family as: 'those related through committed hetero-sexual or same sex partnerships, birth and adoption, and others who have strong emotional and social bonds with a patient' (2004: 155).

KEY POINTS

- During palliative care most care giving is provided by family members and those in close social and emotional relationships.
- Caring for a dying family member is unpredictable and uncertain in duration and nature.
- Family carers are central to the achievement of care preferences in the final phases of life, especially when palliative care and dying are conducted at home.
- Family carers provide a substantial but largely hidden contribution to palliative care.
- Most family care, to those near the end of life is provided by women, spouses and by those in the same generation, and most carers will themselves be older people.
- The impact of care giving is mixed with positive benefits including greater emotional closeness, satisfaction from fulfilling one's duty, and negative effects including increased risk of physical illness and injury, psychological distress, social isolation, financial and employment constraints. While some effects are felt only at the time of caregiving, others, such as financial loss, may have long-term consequences.
- Assessment of caregiving should examine both positive aspects and demands.
- There are three models underpinning supportive interventions: 'burden model', 'stress and coping' and a 'social' model.
- Supportive interventions may be targeted directly at carers or indirectly via support to patients. They include three broad groups of support: education and information provision, social support and therapeutic support.

DISCUSSION

Caring is fundamental to human survival and throughout the life span, people care about and for others; both within and outside family and kinship groups. Some people take on this role suddenly, and it may only last just a few weeks or months as a relative enters the dying phase of a final illness, while for others it lasts a long time with more uncertainty about dying, such as for an older person with dementia. Most carers manage very well and draw upon the support of family members and wider social networks. They may not identify with the term 'carers', as the caregiving role is regarded as part of the normal complex pattern of reciprocal relationships that are characteristic of most family, kinship and friendship systems. Most caregiving is enmeshed in a web of mutual dependencies, responsibilities, demands and rewards that make up everyday family life. Care giving within palliative care contexts, arguably, is especially demanding because of the sense of imminent loss and the demands of caring for a patient with high dependency needs (Payne and Hudson, 2009).

It is difficult to estimate exactly how many people are engaged in caring for a person near the end of life but within Europe there are estimated to be 100 million carers with an estimated 500,000 people providing such care in the UK. Their contribution to care often exceeds the financial expenditures of their countries on formal nursing services. While we know little about the numbers of people who provide care for dying people, we know that caregiving is a gendered role, with care predominantly provided by women and that the majority of carers are in the age range 50–59 but increasingly older people over 65 years are involved in caring both for their spouse and parents who may now live into late old age (over 85 years). In palliative care, there is more likely to be within-generational than cross-generational care giving, which is different from other types of caring. It is often not acknowledged that children may be both the receivers and providers of care within palliative care. Informal, unpaid care giving is largely hidden and taken for granted but it is crucially important to enabling dying people to achieve a 'good death' and in saving society from the huge costs of institutional care (Gomes and Higginson, 2006). Hospice and palliative care services generally recognise the important role that family carers play in providing care and support to patients.

Effects on carers

When a family member becomes seriously ill, care giving involves emotional and psychosocial support as well as the provision of physical care. There is already considerable research identifying the needs of carers in palliative care situations. The evidence includes needs for: psychological support, information, help with domestic tasks, personal care, nursing and medical care of the cared-for person, respite, social and financial help (Hudson and Payne, 2008). There is also a lot of research into the negative effects of care giving, such as anxiety, depression, stress, strain, fatigue and even increased mortality (Grande et al., 2009). Caring for a terminally ill person places heavy financial demands upon the family. The costs of providing medical care, transport to hospital appointments, additional equipment or home adaptations, laundry, heating, clothing and special food are rarely acknowledged. Much of the early literature concentrated on the negative impact, more recently there has been greater recognition of the rewarding aspects of care giving such as closer relationships, feelings of self-esteem and discharging family obligations.

Models of care giving

The 'burden' model focuses on the challenges and problems of being a care giver. Caring is measured in terms of tasks (mainly physical, nursing or domestic roles). The impact of caring is measured in terms of individual deficits such as loss of health (back injuries, depression), income, employment and opportunities for social engagement. It construes carers as overburdened by tasks of caring and there is little recognition of the positive aspects of care.

The 'stress and coping' model emphasizes the thoughts and 'coping' abilities of individual carers which explains why there are such different responses to being a carer.

The 'social' model sees carers as citizens with rights and responsibilities which raises important challenges for public policy, the economy and the wider society. Care giving is seen as being embedded within existing social and family relationships, dependencies and dominance hierarchies such as the role of women in society. Carers are seen as resilient and remarkable people because most manage the role with little formal acknowledgement or financial support (Payne, 2007).

Assessment

It has been recommended that family carers are offered assessment of their own needs at regular intervals (NICE, 2004). There are a number of ways to identify these needs but none is perfect (Payne and Hudson, 2008; Help the Hospices, 2009).

Supportive interventions

A review has shown that while there are lots of different types of support services for carers, there is no strong evidence about which type of support is best (Harding and Higginson, 2003). Table 4.1 offers a framework for understanding that interventions can be targeted directly at carers or have indirect benefit by supporting patients, and that supportive inventions can be clustered into three overlapping groups.

PRACTICAL APPLICATION OF THE CONCEPT

Insights in the words of carers

I think my mum is dying, or it is the beginning of the end. My mum is 89. I just want her to have a quiet, peaceful, pain-free, dignified death – that's what I want for my mum. They said there had been a very severe bleed and they were not expecting her to recover. It was handled very calmly and very sensitively.

(Daughter talking about her mother dying following a stroke)

This quotation highlights that care giving can take the form of concerns and emotional expression in the face of approaching death. It is an example of dying in a hospital where sensitive and compassionate communication has helped this family member to realise what is happening. It also demonstrates the preferences that this person has for a 'good death'.

He's supposed to be my main carer but at the moment I think it's me looking after him more than the other way round.

(Female patient, aged 71, carer is spouse, aged 79)

In a study of the palliative care needs of older people with heart failure living at home, the interdependencies of a frail older couple are revealed (Barnes et al., 2006) in this quotation.

Table 4.1 Framework of intention of supportive interventions for family carers

	Information/Education/Training	Social support	Therapeutic support
Interventions directed at carers	Information on: Care-giving role Bereavement/grief Grants, budgeting and financial management Moving and handling Symptom management Preparing for patient's death	Drop-in centres Lunch clubs Walking groups Help securing grants and welfare benefits	Counselling Complementary therapies Therapeutic groups
Interventions directed at patients that have secondary benefit for carers	Information on: Disease process Managing symptoms Self care strategies Healthy eating and relaxation	Respite Day care In-home sitting services	Counselling Complementary therapies Physiotherapy Occupational therapy

Source: Payne and Hudson (2009)

See also: *caring for the older person; communication; financial aspects for patients and carers; good death*

FURTHER READING

Help the Hospices (2009) *Identifying Carers' Needs in the Palliative Care Setting.* London: Help the Hospices.

Hudson, P. and Payne, S. (eds) (2008) *Family Carers and Palliative Care.* Oxford: Oxford University Press.

REFERENCES

Barnes, S., Gott, M., Payne, S., Parker, C., Seamark, D., Gariballa, S. and Small, N. (2006) 'Characteristics and views of family carers in older people with heart failure', *International Journal of Palliative Nursing*, 12(8): 380–9.

Gomes, B. and Higginson, I. (2006) 'Factors influencing death at home in terminally ill patients with cancer: a systematic review', *British Medical Journal*, 332: 515–21.

Grande, G., Stajduhar, K., Aoun, S., Toye, C., Funk, L., Addington-Hall, J., Payne, S. and Todd, C. (2009). 'Supporting lay carers in end of life care: current gaps and future priorities', *Palliative Medicine*, 23(4): 339–44.

Harding, R. and Higginson, I. (2003) 'What is the best way to help caregivers in cancer and palliative care? A systematic literature review of interventions and their effectiveness', *Palliative Medicine*, 17(1): 63–74.

Help the Hospices (2009) *Identifying Carers' Needs in the Palliative Care Setting*. London: Help the Hospices.

Hudson, P. and Payne, S. (eds) (2008) *Family Carers and Palliative Care*. Oxford: Oxford University Press.

National Institute for Health and Clinical Excellence (NICE) (2004) 'Services for families and carers, including bereavement care', in *Improving Supportive and Palliative Care for Adults with Cancer: The Manual*. London: National Institute for Clinical Excellence.

Payne, S. (2007) 'Resilient carers and caregivers', in B. Monroe and D. Oliviere (eds), *Resilience in Palliative Care: Achievement in Adversity*. Oxford: Oxford University Press, pp. 83–97.

Payne, S. and Hudson, P. (2008) 'Family carers', in D. Walsh, A. Caraceni, K. Foley, R. Fainsinger, C. Goh, P. Glare, M. Lloyd-Williams, J. Nunez Olarte and L. Radbruch (eds), *Palliative Medicine*. New York: Elsevier.

Payne, S. and Hudson, P. (2009) 'European Association for Palliative Care Task Force on Family Carers: aims and objectives', *European Journal of Palliative Care*, 16(2): 77–81.

5 caring for the child with palliative care needs

Yvonne Flood

DEFINITION

The World Health Organisation (WHO, 1998) identified children's palliative care as an active and holistic process involving the child and the family. It should begin on diagnosis and the focus should be on the alleviation of the child's physical, psychological and social distress. Care can be provided in a variety of settings including, home, hospice or hospital and requires a broad multidisciplinary approach. Children's palliative care is a relatively new and developing speciality and while the principles of palliative care for children and adults have many similarities, there are many ways in which they are different. While adult palliative care is often focused on cancer, children with palliative care needs have a wide range of conditions that may be life-threatening or life-limiting. Life-limiting conditions are those from which 'there is no reasonable hope of cure and from which children and young people may die' (ACT/RCPCH, 2003). Life-threatening conditions are those for which 'curative treatment may be feasible but can fail, such as cancer' (ACT/RCPCH, 2003). Children's palliative care is defined by the Association for Children's Palliative Care (ACT) and the Royal College of Paediatrics and Child Health (RCPCH) as 'an active and total approach to care, embracing physical, emotional, social and spiritual elements. It focuses on enhancements of quality of life for the child and support for the family, and includes the management of distressing symptoms provision of respite and care through death and bereavement' (ACT/RCPCH, 2003).

The Children Act (Department of Health, 1989) defines children as those up to the age of 18 years. While chronological age may not necessarily correlate to intellectual age, the needs of young people and children are frequently divided within care provision in children's services. ACT (2001) identifies young people as those between 13 and 24 and therefore for the purpose of this chapter the terms child and children will specifically refer to children aged 12 years and under.

KEY POINTS

Utilising the ACT and WHO definitions, three key issues in palliative care for children will be explored:

- the nature of palliative care for children;
- meeting the needs of the child;
- the role of the multidisciplinary team.

DISCUSSION

The nature of palliative care for children

Palliative care services for children began in the 1980s and the first children's hospice, Helen House, opened in 1982 providing home-from-home care to children with life-limiting illness, and services have continued to develop over the past 27 years. Service provision has often been unplanned and is heavily reliant on voluntary contributions. A recent review of palliative care services identifies children's palliative care as having 'Cinderella status' and goes on to suggest that a lack of understanding may have contributed to this with 'most assuming it is just about end of life care' (Craft and Killen, 2007: 13).

It has been estimated that 20,100 children between 0–19 are likely to require access to palliative care services annually (18,000 if neonatal deaths are excluded). At strategic health authority level, that equates to between 900–2,600 children between 0–19 who will require palliative care services (Department of Health, 2007). While overall the numbers are small in comparison to adult services, children requiring palliative care have a wide range of conditions, some of which are often rare, this makes it difficult to predict and define care needs (Department of Health, 2008).

In order to facilitate the development of services, conditions have been categorised into four broad groups (ACT/RCPCH, 2003):

- Conditions for which curative treatment may be feasible but can fail and where access to palliative care may be necessary when treatment fails e.g. leukaemia, irreversible organ failure.
- Conditions where premature death is inevitable but where periods of invasive treatment may prolong and improve the quality of life.
- Progressive conditions where treatment is exclusively palliative and may extend for many years, e.g. mucopolysaccharidoses, muscular dystrophy.
- Irreversible non-progressive conditions causing severe disability leading to susceptibility to health complications and the likelihood of premature death e.g. severe cerebral palsy.

It is essential that children's palliative care starts at diagnosis and this can mean that the palliative care phase for children can often be long and unpredictable with children requiring frequent medical intervention. Conditions are often familial and may affect more than one child. Many children with palliative care needs have severe disability and while they may not be receiving treatment, are at high risk of complications which may lead to death but may live for many years. This can lead to difficulty in identifying the move to exclusively palliative care and is a challenge to services (Watson et al., 2005: 443).

Meeting the needs of the child

Better Care: Better Lives, the first ever strategy for children's palliative care, states in its vision that services should be 'responsive and respectful to the diverse needs of children' and that children should be enabled to 'fulfill their potential irrespective of their circumstances' (Department of Health, 2008). The ACT (ACT/RCPCH, 2003) definition identifies the requirement to meet the physical, emotional, social and spiritual needs of the child and in order to do this practitioners must have an understanding of developmental, educational and family issues that will impact on the individual child. Major developmental changes occur in infancy and childhood and are concerned with, physical, cognitive, emotional and social development.

Cognitive development is related to the children's understanding of the world around them and their place in it. As their cognitive and emotional understanding develops, so does their understanding of illness and death. The relationship between development and illness is a 'bidirectional' one (Watson et al., 2005: 446) in that the child's development can impact on the child's experience and understanding of the illness and the illness itself can impact on the child's development. Children who have a long-term or chronic illness can develop sophisticated levels of understanding (Watson et al., 2005: 446). This can be a challenge to families, and to those working with them, as their natural desire to protect children conflicts with the child's increasing need for autonomy. Children, where possible, should be involved in the decision-making process and empowered to express their wishes and fears. Communication is a vital aspect of this process and professionals must communicate with children in a way that reflects their level and capacity of understanding. Many children with palliative care needs are unable to express their needs verbally and methods for non-verbal communication should be available.

As school-age children strive to develop their independence, their relationship with their peers becomes ever more important. School is an essential part of the child's day and contributes to children's social well-being as well as their education. Attendance at school enables children to continue their peer relationships and enables ongoing connection with their normal world. All schools must now have special educational needs policies which identify the arrangements to meet special health care needs (ACT/RCPCH 2003).

'One of the most difficult things a parent has to face is being told that their child is likely to die before they will' (Department of Health, 2008). The families of children with palliative care needs and, in particular parents, frequently take on the responsibility for the child's daily care, and in many cases provide highly technical care. Practitioners must be aware of the possible impact on various aspects of family life, such as roles, relationships and financial burden and there is a need for flexible short break provision. It is vital that those working with the child and family work within the philosophy of partnership, families are the experts in their own child's needs and condition. Consideration must also be given to the needs of siblings, who may manifest a range of emotions and behaviour, and time given to the sick child limits the parents' ability to spend time with them. In common with their sick sibling, their physical, cognitive, emotional and social development will impact on their experience and understanding.

The physiological development has a direct relationship with pharmacokinetics and children's ability to metabolise and utilise medications is related to their physiological maturity. This, combined with rarity of some conditions, can make symptom control a challenge. It is important to adopt an individualised approach that takes into account the specific needs of the child and their family.

Multidisciplinary child-centred approaches

A child with life-limiting and life-threatening conditions receives services from a wide range of agencies, including health, education, social care and the private and voluntary sectors. Evidence would suggest that this can at times be fragmented and uncoordinated leading to poor outcomes (Department of Health, 2007).

The National Service Framework Standard 8 (Department of Health and Department for Education and Skills, 2004) states that a multidisciplinary child-centred approach is required and recommends 'a range of flexible sensitive services should be put into place to take account of the physical, practical and emotional needs of the child with a life-limiting illness and their family'. The association for children with life-limiting and life-threatening conditions (ACT) has developed an integrated multiagency care pathway to facilitate the linking of children and families with community services, hospital services, social services, education and the voluntary sector (ACT/RCPCH 2004). The pathway is divided into three sections relating to a particular stage in the child's life, diagnosis, living with a life-limiting illness and end of life and bereavement care. In order to ensure effective coordination of care it is recommended that a key worker is identified (ACT/RCPCH 2004; Department of Health, 2008). The national strategy for children with palliative care needs *Better Care, Better Lives* (Department of Health, 2008), sets out a clear framework for all partners to work together to improve the health and well-being and experiences of services with child and family at the centre of delivery. It is also important that professionals themselves are supported as this may be an unfamiliar area of practice.

PRACTICAL APPLICATION OF THE CONCEPT

Samantha is 8 years old. She lives at home with her parents and her two sisters. Samantha was diagnosed with infantile spasms during the first 12 months of life. Subsequent investigation identified spastic quadriplegia and developmental delay. Samantha has frequent admissions to the local paediatric unit with respiratory infections usually during the winter months. Samantha is no longer able to take sufficient nutrition orally and has had a percuntaneous endoscopic gastrostomy inserted. Samantha's parents provide the majority of her care and her mum has recently given up her job as Samantha's condition has become less stable. Samantha attends a special needs school in the area but as it is not local she is taken there on a daily basis by the school transport. The local children's community nursing team support Samantha at home and act as the key worker, coordinating and liaising with the agencies that are involved in providing services for Samantha and her family. Samantha's two sisters attend the local young carers group. Samantha enjoys her short breaks at the children's hospice and Samantha's parents welcome the opportunity to spend time with their other daughters.

See also: *agencies; caring for the carers; caring for young people; death*

FURTHER READING

Bee, H. (2000) *The Developing Child*. Boston, MA: Allyn and Bacon.
Goldman, A., Hain, R. and Liben, S. (2006) *Oxford Textbook of Palliative Care for Children*. Oxford: Oxford University Press.

caring for the child

REFERENCES

Association for Children with Life-threatening or Terminal Conditions and their Families (ACT) (2001) *Palliative Care for Young People 13–24: Report of the Joint Working Party of ACT, National Council for Hospice and Specialist Palliative Care Services and Scottish Partnership Agency for Palliative and Cancer Care*. Bristol: ACT.

Association for Children with Life-threatening or Terminal Conditions and their Families and The Royal College of Paediatrics and Child Health (ACT/RCPCH) (2003) *A Guide to the Development of Palliative Care Services*. Bristol: ACT/RCPCH.

Association for Children with Life-threatening or Terminal Conditions and their Families and The Royal College of Paediatrics and Child Health (ACT/RCPCH) (2004) *Integrated Multi-agency Care Pathways for children with Life-threatening and Life-limiting Conditions*. Bristol: ACT/RCPCH.

Craft, A. and Killen, S. (2007) *Palliative Care Services for Children and Young People in England: An Independent Review for the Secretary of State by Professor Sir Alan Craft and Sue Killen*. London: DH Publication.

Department of Health (1989) *Children Act*. London: HMSO.

Department of Health (2007) *Palliative Care Statistics for Children and Young Adults*. London: DH Publications.

Department of Health (2008) *Better Care, Better Lives: Improving Outcomes for Children, Young People and their Families Living with Life Limiting and Life Threatening Illness*. London: DH Publications.

Department of Health and Department for Education and Skills (2004) *National Service Framework for Children, Young People and Maternity Services: Disabled Children and Young People and Those with Complex Needs*. London: DH Publications.

Watson, M., Lucas, C., Hoy, A. and Back, I. (2005) *Oxford Handbook of Palliative Care*. Oxford: Oxford University Press.

World Health Organisation (1998) *Cancer Pain Relief and Palliative Care in Children*. Geneva: WHO.

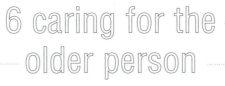

6 caring for the older person

Victoria Ridgway

DEFINITION

Caring for the older person in need of palliative care is a complex process with many pertinent issues in need of addressing, and is too complicated to be defined in simple terms. Palliative care has mainly concentrated on those individuals with cancer and has been successful in reducing suffering towards the end of life. Palliative care now needs to be an integral part of health and social care services providing care for the older person. Currently little research has been carried out on older person's palliative care needs.

KEY POINTS

- An ageing population has a greater demand for palliative care services.
- Many older people have complex problems and disability.
- Caring for the older person requires person-centred care and individual choice.

DISCUSSION

More people are dying of chronic illness than acute, and as the population ages, more individuals in old age will need palliative care services. Twenty per cent of the population are over 65 years of age, with the main causes of death being ischaemic heart disease, cerebro-vascular disease, chronic obstructive pulmonary disease (COPD) and lung cancer (Office of National Statistics, 2008). Of all cancer deaths three-quarters are those aged 65 and above. With the ageing population there will be fewer informal caregivers, increasing the need for health and social care services. Therefore palliative care provision needs to be adapted and developed for the older person. However, older people in England and Wales are under-represented in in-patient hospice care and with increasing age are less likely to receive care for their final illness (World Health Organisation, 2004). Coupled with this, there appears to be a lack of palliative care services in nursing and residential homes, but it could be argued that these individuals receive care according to need.

Older people are more likely to have complex problems, multiple diseases and disabilities, therefore they need packages of care that require collaboration from the inter-professional team. WHO (2004) recommends that because it is difficult to predict the course of chronic disease, for example, exacerbations and acute on chronic illness, palliative care should be based on patient and family needs and not on prognosis.

Carers

The burden of care on the family has been documented, leading to conflicting emotions and fatigue for the carer (Aldred et al., 2005). Overall, patients with a diagnosis other than cancer are more likely to be cared for by relatives (Addington-Hall and Karlsen, 1999) with much of the time given to care being unpaid and unsupported and, therefore, may affect the well-being of the care givers. Indeed, research by Grov and Eklund (2008) found that care givers are often very vulnerable. Older people want to die at home, however, families are often unprepared for the intensity of care giving (Ross et al.,

2000). Of particular note is the burden on the family in caring for those with dementia and heart failure. This is supported by Aldred et al. (2005) who identified that heart failure affected all aspects of the patient's and carer's lives, reducing social interaction, and leading to isolation. In addition only 1% of hospice in-patients' primary diagnosis is dementia and it is now recommended that care of clients with dementia should be merged with elements of palliative care to provide person-centred care. Thus support is provided for the client in their end of life experience and those caring for them (Kydd et al., 2009).

Involvement in decision-making and knowledge of disease

Knowledge and understanding of disease and prognosis are other areas that necessitate attention for older people requiring palliative care. Those individuals with heart failure, and their families, report uncoordinated care and lack of open communication between professionals that hinder care management. Indeed, lack of professional input is highlighted in Aldred et al.'s (2005) research, coupled with confusion regarding diagnosis. However, this is a common theme in care of the older person with clients asking for more information and to be involved in decision-making.

Ageism in healthcare services

Many older people are marginalised and do not receive information about the full range of services or options available. The term 'a Cinderella service' has been coined with older people being discriminated on the grounds of age. There are numerous examples of ageism in health care, some of which are cited by Help the Aged. Ageism, consequently, is highlighted in the National Service framework for the Older Person standards on person-centred care and discrimination (Department of Health, 2001).

Symptom management

Symptom management (shortness of breath, pain, depression, confusion, constipation, malnutrition, fatigue and generalised weakness) and common problems in old age (risk of falls and reduced mobility, confusion, skin integrity, continence issues, visual and hearing impairments, poly pharmacy) are important needs to be addressed and should be an integral part of any assessment. The single assessment process documentation for the older person addresses a range of these issues (Department of Health, 2001), however, this is not widely used. Patients in old age are more likely than patients with a non-cancer diagnosis to experience pain, nausea and vomiting, a dry mouth, loss of appetite, difficulty swallowing, and pressure ulcers. Those with a non-cancer diagnosis tend to experience fewer distressing symptoms but these are longer-lasting and poorly controlled and will require help or support for longer periods of time. Older people with dementia, however, tend to receive sub-optimal end of life care with inadequate management of symptoms (Chatterjee, 2008), common themes include poor or no pain control, and poorly managed behavioural and psychological symptoms, including hallucinations, depression, agitation and paranoia. Chatterjee goes on to highlight dysphagia, causing aspiration pneumonia, and immobility and incontinence causing urinary tract infections, as common reasons for hospital admissions in end of life care for people with dementia, indeed, 67% of patients with dementia were hospitalised in their last year of life.

Medicine management and pain control

Older people are more prone to adverse drug reactions and have poorer pain management. Approximately a fifth of older people find pain bad enough to limit daily activities, however, older people generally under-report pain, therefore it goes untreated (Age Concern, 2008). Furthermore those with dementia are at risk of receiving no pain management strategies due to underestimation by healthcare staff, and clients' communication problems. However, this underestimation of pain by healthcare professionals occurs across the spectrum of care of the older person. Kydd et al. (2009) suggest that pain management is an area that palliative care services could promote for the older person, adding that expertise in pain control by palliative care teams would help resolve unrelieved pain symptoms that the older person experiences.

End of life care

An aspect that does need consideration is the client's preference for where care is delivered and where death occurs. Currently most older people, those aged over 65, die in acute settings (59%) or long-term care facilities (19%), only 4% die in a hospice and 16% die at home (Age Concern, 2008). However, 75% of older people generally would prefer to be cared for, and die, at home (WHO, 2004). Therefore it could be suggested that the end of life care needs of older people are not adequately addressed.

Sociologically older people are more likely to live alone, experience economic hardship, and be lonely and isolated. The psychological impact of a chronic disease also needs attention, relatives in receipt of specialist palliative care services report fewer psychological symptoms and unmet needs, however, as already discussed, the majority of older people are not cared for in this environment. Older people will also have a heightened awareness that death is drawing closer, and may fear for the future. Common concerns include safety, being able to die with dignity, not dying alone and being prepared for death.

For these reasons, holistic care of the older person should be promoted in end of life care. Age Concern (1999) highlight 12 principles of a good death with the key theme being that of control for the older person in decision-making. Other aspects include spiritual and psychosocial support, the use of complementary therapies, to have physical needs addressed including pain and symptom control. Additionally, there are aspects relating to privacy and dignity, support and the family and care givers, access to specialist palliative care teams and/or non-cancer patient teams, time to say goodbye and, finally, bereavement support.

CONCLUSION

Following the review of current literature on caring for the older person with palliative care needs, it appears that there are several key issues to be addressed to enhance care. These are good pain management, good communication between professional groups and between family/client and professionals, and coordinated team work. Therefore palliative care needs a multifaceted approach to meet the needs of the older person with a life-limiting condition. Addington-Hall and Karlsen (1999) suggest that these older people need a different approach to traditional hospice care, drawing on the principles of autonomy and dignity. Therefore it is up to healthcare professionals to ensure that a palliative care approach is incorporated into care of the older person with a life-limiting condition.

Current work by Age Concern and the National Council for Palliative Care to develop policy and practice in this area will improve quality of care for the older person.

PRACTICAL APPLICATION OF THE CONCEPT

Robert is an 84-year-old gentleman who has been to his GP five times in the last two months with uncontrolled pain in his chest and shoulder. The pain is such that now he is unable to drive his car and maintain his independence, relying on his wife Ellen to care for him. Ellen is finding it difficult to cope and care for Robert. On each visit to the GP Robert's analgesic is altered, from cocodamol to morphine sulphate, this makes Robert drowsy, causing him to fall. He is admitted to hospital, on examination, he is confused, dehydrated, constipated and in pain. He undergoes intensive investigations (scan, blood analysis) and a shadow on his lung is identified. Robert dies two days later on an acute surgical ward, alone.

See also: *cultural issues in palliative care; palliative care and the person with non-cancer diagnosis; policy drivers*

FURTHER READING

Age Concern (2008) 'Policy position papers: death and dying'. Available at: www.agecon-cern.org.uk

Help the Aged (2008) *Worth Fighting For: Ten Stories of Ageism*. London: Help the Aged. Available at: www.helptheaged.org.uk/justequaltreatment

key concepts in
palliative care

World Health Organisation Europe (2004) 'Better palliative care for older people'. Available at: www.euro.who.int/document/E82933.pdf

REFERENCES

Addington-Hall, J.M. and Karlsen, S. (1999) 'Age is not the crucial factor in determining how the palliative care needs of people who die from cancer differ from those of people who die from other causes', *Journal of Palliative Care*, 15(4): 13–19.

Age Concern (1999) *Debate of the Age Health and Social Study Group: The Future of Health and Care of the Older Person. The Best is Yet to Come*. London: Age Concern.

Age Concern (2008) 'Policy position papers: death and dying', available at: www.age concern.org.uk accessed 12 June 2009.

Aldred, H., Gott, M. and Gariballa, S. (2005) 'Advanced heart failure: impact on older patients and informal carers', *Journal of Advanced Nursing*, 49(2): 116–24.

Chatterjee, J. (2008) 'End of life care for patients with dementia', *Nursing Older People*, 20(2): 29–34.

Department of Health (2001) *National Service Framework for Older People: Executive Summary*. London: HMSO.

Grov, E.K. and Eklund, M.L. (2008) 'Reactions of primary caregivers of frail older people and people with cancer in the palliative phase living at home', *Journal of Advanced Nursing*, 63(6): 576–85.

Kydd, A., Duffy, T. and Duffy, F.J.R. (2009) *The Care and Wellbeing of Older People*. Devon: Reflect Press.

Office of National Statistics (2008) Website: www.statistics.gov.uk/cci/nugget.asp?id=1332 accessed 12 June 2009.

Ross, M.M., Fisher, R. and Maclean, M.J. (2000) 'End of life care for seniors: the develop-ment of a national guide', *Journal of Palliative Care*, 16(4): 47–53.

World Health Organisation (WHO) Europe (2004) 'Better palliative care for older people', available at: www.euro.who.int/document/E82933.pdf accessed 12 June 2009.

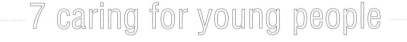

7 caring for young people

Amanda Humphreys and Pat Rose

DEFINITION

The Association for Children with Life-Threatening or Terminal Conditions and their Families (ACT, 2008: 1) defines children's palliative care as 'an active and total approach to care embracing physical, emotional and spiritual elements. It focuses on enhancement of quality of life for the child and support for the whole family and includes the management of distressing symptoms, provision of respite and care from diagnosis through death and bereavement', and defines children as young people up to the age of 18 years. However, the Teenage Cancer Trust (TCT, 2009) suggests the age range of 13 and 24 years as the definition of young people. This chapter will use the ACT definition but substitutes the term 'young person' for child and defines young people as aged 13 to 24 years. This age range crosses the boundary between paediatric and adult services and can therefore impact on service provision to this group.

KEY POINTS

- Family dynamics change when a young person is life-limited.
- A range of losses are experienced by all family members.
- The transition between paediatric and adult services is a difficult time.

DISCUSSION

Changing family dynamics

While a young person would naturally move from being dependent to independent, throughout the trajectory from diagnosis through life-limiting illness the young person is faced with a heightened reliance on parents and carers which is in direct conflict with the adolescent's developmental tasks of gaining independence and autonomy (Smith et al., 2007). Within this return to dependency there is the specific intrusion regarding personal matters, for example, bathing and toileting. This invasion of privacy can hamper family relationships and initiate conflict. The young person may demonstrate regression and adopt safe, familiar, childlike behaviour. Conversely, the young person may overprotect, and make allowances for, parents by refusing their help. This role reversal may impact on the young person's ability to access support within the family and make them feel rejected. A reciprocal desire to protect the family and young person can result in communication being difficult as each family member can inadvertently collude to avoid confronting the possible death of the young person. The fear of upsetting those close to them can result in the young person not sharing their thoughts and feelings, compounding the perception of isolation. Schultz (2007) suggests the family context has an important influence on the process of identity development for adolescents; therefore stability of relationships is important at this time when the future is in doubt.

As the focus of attention is on the sick young person, the siblings can experience loss of identity and insecurity within the family as well as experiencing a sense of loss about their involvement in care delivery. Rowse (2006) demonstrated that siblings of young people with life-limiting illness can mimic the experience of the young person: isolation, separation and limited sharing of feelings with parents were all identified in some siblings.

Grandparents, while experiencing the intense emotional response to the grandchild's illness will also be affected by their own child's (the parent) distress, as there is an innate urge as a parent to protect your child from distress. Many grandparents help to look after other grandchildren as a result of the child's illness and this may have a huge impact on their daily lives. However, the focus of support by healthcare professionals is often directed solely at the parents (Nehari et al., 2007).

The palliative care team should focus on holistic care of the whole family including ongoing assessment of relationships which is vital for proactive planning, care delivery and evaluation of strategies implemented. Maynard, Rennie, Shirtliffe and Vickers (2005) recognise the service is multi-faceted in providing supportive care, respite, end of life care, information, family support and social activities. As a young person can move in and out of meeting the criteria for additional services, the palliative care team is the constant in the family's life.

The experience of loss

While the ultimate loss is death, Woodgate (2006) identified that families can experience a range of losses while the young person is ill: loss of daily routine, friends, health or income. However, the impact of a diagnosis of life-limiting illness on the young person can be devastating and subsequent treatment can facilitate development of 'accelerated maturity' whereby the young person is catapulted into making complex decisions, or 'delayed youth' whereby the young person is unable to participate in activities with friends (Whiteson, 2003). This can render the young person feeling isolated. Indeed, isolation can be self-induced by a withdrawal from socialising and participating in life experiences. This can be perceived as a protective mechanism and further implies the adolescent's vulnerability, loss of identity, lack of confidence and loss of self-esteem.

Young people gradually relocate from being family-centred towards peer involvement. Identification and acceptance by friends are essential, however, continuity of peer relationships is hampered by the disruptions caused by care delivery. For the young person it can be perceived that 'time stands still', however, their peer group moves on (Smith et al., 2007). This perception can be mirrored by parents as they experience a loss of increasing independence and can perceive that their lives have also been put on hold.

Care delivery can disrupt educational programmes and permanently damage career prospects highlighting loss of a clear career pathway and absence from work. The young person can also perceive loss of their place of refuge, their home, as specialist care, family counselling and technology invade their space. This loss of control can exacerbate conflict within the family.

Transitional care

Whiteson (2003) noted that transition from paediatric to adult services may be delayed because of unwillingness by healthcare professionals to refer onwards, reluctance of the young person and family to leave their familiar support and in recognition of potential 'culture shock'. With the change of environment, the young person can encounter a sense of loss from the established relationships formed within a paediatric setting and will need to establish a new rapport with new people before confiding personal thoughts and feelings. This can take energy at a time when the young person is depleted.

Within the adult environment, there may be a propensity to reflect on childhood experiences and redefine the roles and goals that the new care environment dictates. In the paediatric environment there is a clear partnership between parent and child in decision-making, however, in the adult setting, people are deemed competent to make their own decisions. The young person may well have a reasoned understanding of the illness and the implications, but not necessarily the psychological resources to deal with it. The young person requires a safe arena to express intense emotional responses to the diagnosis as well as opportunities to engage in normal adolescent activities, thus promoting normality at a time when there is limited control over treatment and management of the illness. Hollis and Morgan (2001) propose that adolescents who perceive some sense of control over their treatment and take some responsibility for themselves are more likely to comply with therapy. However, active participation in care delivery and decision-making can be compromised unless sufficient age-appropriate information is provided. Monterosso and Kristjanson (2008) acknowledged the sense of apprehension and uncertainty experienced by parents throughout their child's illness, and yet transitional care can shift from a family-centred approach to an adult one-to-one approach (Miles et al., 2004).

PRACTICAL APPLICATION OF THE CONCEPT

This brief scenario demonstrates the impact of diagnosis on the whole family and the inherent tensions that can erupt and the role of the palliative care team in providing support.

David, aged 15 years, has non-Hodgkin's lymphoma. The family consists of Mum, a teacher, Dad, an accountant, and a younger brother John aged 12 years. The paternal grandfather lives locally. Prior to diagnosis, both brothers played football in a Sunday league while Mum went to church. Recently Mum has stopped David playing football as she feels he is not well enough and she wants the family to start going to church together. David feels isolated from his friends and a burden on his brother. He is slamming doors around the house and staying in his bedroom. John will not go to football without David and refuses to go to church. The palliative care nurse works with the whole family to explore and negotiate compromises such as:

- Mum and Dad buy an interactive football game for David and the family to play.
- David is facilitated to access TCT peer support group to talk through his feelings.

- David is allowed to participate in football training, as much as his health status allows, and to attend matches, help with kit and refreshments whenever possible.
- Once a month the whole family, including John, goes to church.
- Once a month grandfather takes John to football while the others go to church.
- Once a month Mum and Dad take John to the football to encourage his progress.
- Once a month John goes to the football with his friends.

By suggesting a package of compromises such as these, the nurse helps the family resolve their difficulties around Sunday activities and all the family get some of what they want.

See also: *caring for the carers; caring for the child with palliative care needs*

FURTHER READING

Brown, E. and Warr, B. (2007) *Supporting the Child and the Family in Paediatric Palliative Care*. London: Jessica Kingsley Publishers.

National Institute of Health and Clinical Excellence (2005) *Improving Outcomes in Children and Young People with Cancer.* London: NICE.

REFERENCES

Association for Children with Life-Threatening or Terminal Conditions and their Families (ACT) (2008) *Children's Palliative Care: Descriptions and Definitions*. Available at: www.act.org.uk/index.php/about-act/definitions.html, accessed 17 March 2009.

Hollis, R. and Morgan, S. (2001) 'The adolescent with cancer – at the edge of no-man's land', *The Lancet Oncology*, 2: 43–8.

Maynard, L., Rennie, T., Shirtliffe, J. and Vickers, D. (2005) 'Seeking and using families' views to shape children's hospice services', *International Journal of Palliative Nursing*, 11(12): 624–30.

Miles, K., Edwards, S. and Clapson, M. (2004) 'Transition from paediatric to adult services: experiences of HIV-positive adolescents', *AIDS CARE*, 16(3): 305–14.

Monterosso, L.J. and Kristjanson (2008) 'Supportive and palliative care needs of families of children who die from cancer: an Australian study', *Palliative Medicine*, 22(1): 59–69.

Nehari, M., Grebler, D. and Toren, A. (2007) 'A voice unheard: grandparents' grief over children who died of cancer', *Mortality*, 12(1): 66–78.

Rowse, V. (2006) 'Home-based palliative care for children', *Paediatric Nursing*, 18(7): 20–4.

Schultz, L.E. (2007) 'The influence of maternal loss on young women's experience of identity development in emerging adulthood', *Death Studies*, 31: 17–43.

Smith, S., Davies, S., Wright, D., Chapman, C. and Whiteson, M. (2007) 'The experiences of teenagers and young adults with cancer: Results of 2004 conference survey', *European Journal of Oncology Nursing*, 11(4): 362–8.

Teenage Cancer Trust (2009) *About TCT: The Facts*. Available at: www.teenagecancertrust.org/about/about.php, accessed 17 March 2009.

Whiteson, M. (2003) 'The Teenage Cancer Trust – advocating a model for teenage cancer services', *European Journal of Cancer*, 39: 2688–93.

Woodgate, R.L. (2006) 'Life is never the same: childhood cancer narratives', *European Journal of Cancer Care*, 15: 8–18.

8 communication

Jan Woodhouse

DEFINITION

A definition of communication that has stood the test of time is that communication is a two-way process that involves a sender and a receiver (Evans, 1986). There are a number of stages that make up the cycle of communication. First, a message is conceived through thought or external stimuli; this is then encoded using verbal or non-verbal language, a picture or in writing; which is then followed by selection of a communication medium, e.g. interview, letter. These are all in the remit of the sender. The receiver then has to decode the message, using their knowledge of language, culture and vocabulary; interpret the message, i.e. give it a meaning, both underlying and explicitly; and, finally, give feedback to the sender, acknowledging the message. It is easy to see effective communication means getting all the stages right and just as easy to see where things may go wrong.

KEY POINTS

- Good communication skills are essential in the palliative care setting.
- Breaking bad news is both a task and a process.
- Disavowal is more commonly encountered than denial.
- Collusion is a protective mechanism but a barrier to open communication.

DISCUSSION

The readiness to communicate is an essential aspect in the palliative care setting. It has been noted that some healthcare professionals may lack confidence in their own communication skills (Chaturvedi et al., 2009) and if this is the case, then avoidance and being at a loss for words may prevail (Gaultier, 2008). This is the last thing that needy patients and relatives want; it is a time that calls for open and honest communication and, as Gaultier (2008: 292) points out, a time to 'listen more and talk less'. The Department of Health's *End of Life Care Strategy* (2008) identifies that open, honest communication is Step 1 in the plan to deliver effective care. The document also notes that it is important to recognise cues that can lead to discussions. Hence those working in palliative care should undertake additional education in communication skills in order to achieve the above.

Essential skills usually fall into breaking bad news, recognising denial and collusion, and picking up on what is important for the patient and their carers (Dunn, 2002; Edwards, 2005; Chaturvedi et al., 2009). All of these aspects have received a lot of attention over the years – focusing on different diseases, different settings and different healthcare professional groups. The skill of breaking bad news, for example, has been largely targeted at medical personnel (Vandekieft, 2001), mainly because they are the group who usually bring together all the results of investigations, to arrive at a diagnosis, treatment plan and prognosis. Vandekieft (2001: 1978) has brought together a range of breaking bad news models to produce an ABCDE model that deals with both the task and the process. The mnemonics stand for:

A: *Advance preparation* – clinical information, room setting, time, privacy, rehearsal of words and phrases, emotional preparation.

B: *Build a therapeutic environment/relationship* – determine what the patient knows and how much they want to know, provision of support (staff and/or other relatives) if patient desires it, introduction of persons present, warn that bad news is coming, use touch appropriately, follow-up appointment.

C: *Communicate well* – ask what the patient or family already knows, be frank but compassionate, avoid jargon and euphemisms, allow for silence and tears, have the patient repeat their understanding of the news, allow for questions, write things down, summarise and make a follow-up plan.

D: *Deal with patient and family's reactions* – assess and respond to the emotional reaction, repeat at each visit, be empathetic, do not argue with or criticise colleagues.

E: *Encourage and validate emotions* – explore what the news means to patients, offer realistic hope, utilise the multi-disciplinary team, take care of the emotions of self and other staff.

communication

37

This last aspect, of taking care of the emotions, may call for a de-brief and responding to 'how did I/you feel' questions as well as getting feedback on the technique. The truly effective communicator is open to constructive criticism and actively seeks comments on their performance; it is not a sign of insecurity but a demonstration of their willingness to learn from unique situations.

It can be seen in the ABCDE model that an allowance is built in at the B level for the prospect of the patient being in denial. Denial was identified by Freud along with the concept of 'disavowal' (Hardy and Kell, 2009). Hardy and Kell (2009: 22) make the distinction between the two by offering Freud's 1927 definitions:

Denial: the repudiation of reality – an entirely unconscious process of repressing or forgetting information we have been given.

Disavowal: allows individuals to accept information they have been given but find ways to minimise its impact.

While the concept of denial is much used in palliative care, the notion of disavowal is not often highlighted and yet, perhaps, it is the phenomenon that is observed more often. The word 'disavowal', however, seems to have fallen out of common usage and consequently 'denial' has been used in its place. Hardy and Kell (2009) state that with disavowal the patient undergoes two-track thinking – where one minute they can cope with the reality of their situation and the next they have escaped into hope or fantasy and undue optimism. Denial, on the other hand, may mean that the patient cannot let the information into their conscious part of the mind and hence they deny knowledge of their condition and will wonder what you are talking about. This, Hardy and Kell point out, is quite a rare state. While it is accepted that denial and disavowal are among several normal coping mechanisms (others Hardy and Kell identify are: secrecy and concealment, illusion of control, minimising/rationalising, pretence/avoidance, and behavioural escape), breaking of them may shatter hope. Hardy and Kell note that it can be a problematic state. However, they ask if it is a problem, then 'who for?', and 'why is it a problem?' Confronting denial and disavowal may be necessary if care is to be executed in the best interests of the patient, e.g. they have to be admitted to a care setting because their caregivers can no longer cope. Hardy and Kell (2009: 24) suggest that it should be 'communicated respectfully and gently, in small manageable chunks, allowing space for them to process and reflect on what they are being told.' From experience, it may be noted that breaking of denial and disavowal may be followed by an emotional response, such as anger and depression.

In order to prevent negative emotions, such as those mentioned above, another phenomenon occurs regularly in the palliative care setting, that of collusion. Chaturvedi et al. (2009) point out that collusion, where information is not shared or is actively withheld between individuals, can differ according to the prevailing culture and the family dynamics. It often appears about the time of delivering a diagnosis and again when there is a move from the curative mode to the palliative mode. It appears to be an unconscious protective mechanism that reduces distress and anxiety for both the patient and their carers. Chaturvedi et al. note that it can result in a 'recovery plot', where the focus is on treatment and positive outcomes rather than addressing the prognosis, increasing dependency, potential symptoms and subsequent death. They comment that the families are more involved in the patient *getting better* rather than *feeling better* (2009: 3). Some reasons given for the emergence of collusion is the emotionality of anticipated loss, a perceived reluctance of healthcare personnel to discuss death and dying, and the superstition that talking about death may hasten the event. Hence it can be seen that collusion can be multi-factorial in its nature. If collusion is allowed to exist, then open communication is reduced and aspects such as dealing with unfinished business, emotional release and future planning may be impaired (Chaturvedi et al., 2009). On the other hand, challenging collusion and gaining open communication may bring with it 'emotional outbursts, despair, demoralisation and depression' (Chaturvedi et al., 2009: 3). It is hardly surprising, then, that healthcare staff may find themselves party to collusion. However, these effects are usually short-term and so open communication should remain the goal of healthcare professionals.

Useful adjuncts to aid healthcare workers in their communication skills are the many talking therapies and other communication models. These are high-lighted in Table 8.1.

Table 8.1   Additional communication models

Model	What it offers
Counselling skills	Emphasis on active listening; Non-judgemental attitude; Giving and receiving feedback: Personal insight
Transactional Analysis (TA)	Recognising parent, adult and child ego states in conversations; Life scripts: The drama triangle (victim, persecutor, rescuer); Positive and negative strokes; Life positions (I'm Okay, You're Okay, etc.)
Neuro-Linguistic Programming	Understanding of the modalities that are used in conversation; Recognising visual cues to thinking; Visual imaging to reduce symptoms
Organisational behaviour	Understanding the concept of group dynamics and power relationships
Cognitive Behavioural Therapy	Changing thinking patterns; Recognising response triggers; Goal-planning
Body language	Understanding and recognising non-verbal language: gestures, sounds and body language
Diagrammatic mapping	Using Genograms – to elicit family trees and patterns of illness and Ecomaps – that help to identify personal relationships and levels of support
Expressive arts	Communication using art, storytelling, poetry, narrative, music, body movement
Dementia awareness	Understanding the confusional state – the use of metaphor, seeing others, premonition
Sign language and picture boards	Enables communication with those with hearing impairment and cognitive impairment

communication

39

PRACTICAL APPLICATION OF THE CONCEPT

Elizabeth was in her seventies, single, lived alone and was dying from uterine cancer. She had been admitted to hospital for symptom control. The consultant told the nursing staff that she probably had another month to live. Elizabeth kept asking when she could go home but the nursing staff kept avoided answering her question. The ward manager made time to sit with Elizabeth and to find out what Elizabeth understood of her condition. Elizabeth replied that she knew that she was dying and that it presented difficulties because she lived on her own but that was where she wanted to be. The ward manager arranged for supportive care to be given to Elizabeth and Elizabeth went home to die. The ward manager faced criticism from some of her colleagues because they felt that the hospital was the better care environment for Elizabeth. However, she was able to justify her decision on the strength of the conversation that she had with Elizabeth and the expressed wishes.

See also: environment of care; sexuality; spirituality

FURTHER READING

Brewin, T. (1996) *Relating to the Relatives: Breaking Bad News, Communication and Support.* Oxford: Radcliffe Medical Press.

Dunn, N. (2002) *Cancer Tales: Communicating in Cancer Care.* London: Haymarket Medical Publications.

Heyse-Moore, L. (2009) *Speaking of Dying: A Practical Guide to Using Counselling Skills in Palliative Care.* London: Jessica Kingsley Publishers.

REFERENCES

Chaturvedi, S.K., Loiselle, C.G. and Chandra, P.S. (2009) 'Communication with relatives and collusion in palliative care: a cross-cultural perspective', *Indian Journal of Palliative Care*, 15(1): 2–9.

Department of Health (2008) *End of Life Care Strategy.* London: DH.

Dunn, N. (2002) *Cancer Tales: Communicating in Cancer Care.* London: Haymarket Medical Publications.

Edwards, P. (2005) 'An overview of the end-of-life discussion', *International Journal of Palliative Nursing*, 11(1): 21–7.

Evans, D.W. (1986) *People, Communication and Organisations.* London: Pitman Publishing.

Gaultier, D.M. (2008) 'Challenges and opportunities: communication near the end of life', *Medsurg Nursing*, 17(5): 291–6.

Hardy, R. and Kell, C. (2009) 'Understanding and working with the concept of denial and its role as a coping strategy', *Nursing Times*, 105(32–3): 22–4.

Vandekieft, G.F. (2001) 'Breaking bad news', *American Family Physician*, 64(12): 1975–8.

9 concept of death

Jill McCarthy

DEFINITION

Death is the departure from life and the permanent end of all physiological functioning. It is a process rather than an event and is normally determined by the irreversible cessation of neural, cardiac and respiratory activity. The Department of Health defines death as 'the irreversible loss of the capacity for consciousness, combined with the irreversible loss of the capacity to breathe' (Department of Health, 2006: 7). With the onset of modern medicine, situations now occur whereby artificial interventions are used to maintain cardiorespiratory functioning and, in these cases, brain function tests are used to determine death. In legislation, there is no statutory definition of death in the United Kingdom at the present time (Department of Health, 2006: 7). Spirituality and religion are both meaningful social constructs which afford a helpful viewpoint from which to consider the subject of death and dying and these can provide comfort and solace to both the terminally ill and those bereaved.

KEY POINTS

- Death is the cessation of physiological functioning.
- Death is a process rather than an event.
- Where cardiorespiratory function is maintained artificially, brain function tests determine death.
- There is no statutory definition of death within British law.
- Death and dying are emotionally laden subjects.

DISCUSSION

On average, half a million people die annually in the United Kingdom (Department of Health, 2007). This is often a particularly distressing time for relatives and friends and it is common for a period of mourning and grieving to follow a death. There is a great mystery surrounding dying and death, particularly as the process has become medicalised within modern society (Illich, 1976). Lay people are now generally removed from caring for a dying relative at home and from paying respects to a neighbour who has died and is laid out in the house, as was commonplace prior to the introduction of the National Health Service in 1948 (Clark, 2002). For many people, the first experience of death and dying is when a relative is seriously ill in a hospital or nursing home, and family members and close friends gather around the bedside in vigil to watch over the person until death occurs.

The hospice movement has brought with it the concepts of palliative care and good death (Saunders, 1981). What constitutes a good death will differ from person to person, but will contain common factors such as: being free from pain and discomfort; dying in a venue of choice, for example, at home or in a hospice; open acknowledgement of the imminence of death; a sense of completion in that tasks are accomplished, goodbyes have been said and a life-review has taken place; and knowledge that loved ones will be taken care of as far as is possible. Few anticipations of a good death would involve dying in a medical setting or being surrounded by healthcare staff and yet, in the United Kingdom, 60% of all deaths still occur in a hospital setting (Clark, 2002).

Death is not always a straightforward issue, however, and it is sometimes difficult to ascertain when a person is deemed to have crossed over from life into death. The criterion by which we mark the death of a person is not always clear-cut and the United Kingdom (unlike the United States of America) lacks legislation to clarify this subject. Prior to the introduction of medical technology, death was commonly ascertained by failure of the cardiopulmonary systems, a comparatively easy assessment. However, since the introduction of medical ventilators and enteral feeding, this definition of death is no longer adequate for some people who are severely brain damaged but supported with the aid of medical technology and artificial feeding. For such people, whose lungs are functioning adequately only through artificial ventilation, the more complex definition of brain stem death has become more appropriate (the brain stem is involved in control of the cardiovascular system, the respiratory system, pain sensitivity, alertness, and consciousness and, thus, brain stem damage is life-threatening). This is in order to allow futile treatments to be withdrawn and organs to be donated, if appropriate, in the full knowledge that the condition of the person concerned could not be improved.

The 'beating heart cadaver', as people in this condition are sometimes referred to (Machado, 2005), present an ethical dilemma in terms of the definition of death. Should brain stem dead patients be regarded as dead or as having a hopeless prognosis? If they are regarded as dead, then it would appear logical that there should be no physical response to stimuli. However, it is necessary to anaesthetise these patients while harvesting organs for transplantation, otherwise blood pressure can rise dramatically when the first incision is made and the brain-dead body can react when nerves are cut, giving the appearance of shrugging, kicking or, perhaps, signalling (Sharp, 2006). Conversely, if they are to be regarded as having a hopeless prognosis, then logic would dictate that they are still alive and, therefore, we have no right to remove organs or turn off life support machines. It would seem, therefore, that there is a difference between the death of a body and the death of a person (Gillet, 1990) and with brain stem death, although the body is still functioning to some extent, it is believed that the actual person had died.

This is an extremely distressing time for the relatives, partners and friends of such patients and it is important that they are kept fully informed in a sympathetic and appropriate manner. To the layperson's eye, their relative may be unconscious, but they are warm to the touch and look healthy with hearts that are beating independently, which is a far cry from the usual criteria for death. This can make it very difficult for some relatives to accept that their loved one had died. Pugh et al. (2000) suggest that it may be pertinent, in some cases, to ask relatives if they would like to be present while the testing for brain stem death takes place, in order to 'improve understanding that death has occurred'. It has been known for some relatives to object strongly to artificial ventilation being discontinued, as they have confused brain stem death with persistent vegetative state, whereby patients have regained consciousness on rare occasions (Pugh et al., 2000).

CONCLUSION

Modern medicine has brought with it many changes, not least the definition of when a person is alive and when they are dead. With artificial ventilation, the body of a person who is brain stem dead can be kept functioning to some degree, although the actual person is no longer alive. This has raised ethical concerns with the public in some quarters, in part because the condition of brain stem death is sometimes confused with persistent vegetative state from which people have been known to recover. However, the medical profession is clear that brain stem death equates with death of a person and, therefore, all treatment should be withdrawn.

PRACTICAL APPLICATION OF THE CONCEPT

David, who was 28 years of age, was involved in a serious road traffic accident. He was transferred to the nearest Accident and Emergency Unit by emergency ambulance, unfortunately his condition continued to deteriorate and he was transferred to the Intensive Care Unit where he was attached to an artificial ventilator. Three days later, two doctors carried out tests for brain stem death and it was confirmed, through the tests, that he had died. David was married with a 2-year-old daughter.

Throughout David's admission and stay in hospital, his wife Sally and his mother and father were kept fully informed by the unit staff of his condition. The day prior to testing for brain stem death, the unit manager sat down with David's family and explained in a sensitive and caring manner exactly what the tests were designed to show and how brain stem death differed from persistent vegetative state. Sally kept stating that she couldn't understand how David might be dead because he looked so well, there were no outward signs of injury and he was warm to touch and she could hear his heart beating when she held him. The unit manager was calm and understanding, repeating the information in order to give the family time to absorb it; aware that it was shocking news that was difficult for them to comprehend at this time.

The following day the family were more prepared for the result of the tests which had diagnosed brain stem death. The manager discussed withdrawal of treatment and advised the family that this could be distressing to witness, but that they would arrange for the family to be present if this was their wish. The family decided that they would say goodbye to David, but that they did not wish to witness the discontinuation of treatment. The subject of organ donation was discussed gently and sensitively by the unit coordinator, but Sally felt that this was not appropriate as David had never talked about this and she considered, without his express permission, that it would be a violation of his body.

See also: *good death; hospice movement and evolution of palliative care; value of life*

FURTHER READING

DeSpelder, L.A. and Strickland, A.L. (2005) *The Last Dance: Encountering Death and Dying*, 6th edn. New York: McGraw-Hill.
Kübler-Ross, E. (1981) *Living with Death and Dying*. London: Souvenir Press.
Kübler-Ross, E. (1986) *Death: The Final Stage of Growth*. New York: Touchstone.

REFERENCES

Clark, D. (2002) 'Between hope and acceptance: the medicalisation of dying', *British Medical Journal*, 324(7342): 905–7.
Department of Health (2006) *Draft for Consultation. Section 1. A Code of Practice for the Diagnosis and Certification of Death*. London: Department of Health.
Department of Health (2007) *Consultation on Improving the Process of Death Certification*. London: Department of Health.
Gillet, G.R. (1990) 'Consciousness, the brain and what matters', *Bioethics*, 4(3): 181–98.
Illich, I. (1976) *Limits to Medicine: Medical Nemesis: The Expropriation of Health*. London: Marion Boyars.
Machado, C. (2005) 'The first organ transplant from a brain-dead donor', *Neurology*, 64: 1938–42.
Pugh, J., Clarke, L., Gray, J., Haveman, J., Lawler, P. and Bonner, S. (2000) 'Presence of relatives during testing for brain stem death: questionnaire study', *British Medical Journal*, 321: 1505–06.
Saunders, C. (1981) *Hospice: The Living Idea*. London: Hodder Arnold.
Sharp, L. (2006) *Strange Harvest*. Berkeley, CA: University of California Press.

10 coronial process

Richard Griffith

DEFINITION

The coroner is one of the oldest judicial offices and is mentioned in the Articles of Ayre of 1194 where the coroners' duties, apart from investigating sudden deaths, also included investigations that could raise money for the Crown. Their role continues today under the provisions of the Coroners Rules 1984 (as amended by the Coroners (Amendment) Rules 2005) and the Coroners Act 1988.

The role of the modern coroner is to hold an inquest where they are informed that the body of a person is lying within their district and there is reasonable cause to suspect that the deceased:

- has died a violent or an unnatural death;
- has died a sudden death of which the cause is unknown; or
- has died in prison or in such a place or in such circumstances as to require an inquest under any other Act.

KEY POINTS

- The coroner is one of the oldest judicial offices in the country.
- The administrative system for registering death relies heavily on the opinion of a doctor to corroborate that a person has died and the coroner oversees and scrutinises this system.
- The duty of the coroners is to inquire into the circumstances and cause of deaths reported to them.
- Where the deceased has a violent or an unnatural death; a sudden death of which the cause is unknown; or has died in prison, the coroner must hold an inquest.

DISCUSSION

The duty of the coroners is to inquire into the circumstances and cause of deaths reported to them. Coroners will establish the identity of the deceased, the circumstances surrounding the death and the medical cause of death. They are assisted in their investigations by the police. Coroners are lawyers or qualified medical practitioners of no less than five years standing (Coroner's Act 1988, section 2). They are appointed by local authorities and their duties are overseen by the Ministry of Justice.

The administrative system for confirming death relies heavily on the opinion of a doctor to corroborate that a person has died. The system requires checks and balances to prevent wrongdoing and there is a duty on the doctor attending the patient during their last illness or who sees the body after death to issue a medical certificate of cause of death. The death must be registered with the Registrar of Births, Marriages and Deaths (Births and Deaths Registration Act 1953 s 22). Where the registrar has the information to complete the entry in the death register and decides that the death does not need reporting to the coroner the registrar will issue;

- a Certificate for Burial or Cremation, and
- a Certificate of Registration of Death required for Social Security purposes, and
- where requested, copies of the entry in the Death Register, usually called the death certificate. Two copies of the death certificate are generally required by the person's representative in order to show banks and insurance companies when settling the person's affairs.

In the case of cremation, the family representative must make an application for cremation and the doctor who provided the medical certificate of cause of death completes the cremation form along with a second doctor, not in the same practice as the first, who has been qualified for more than five years. This second doctor is now required to contact the person caring for the deceased to ask if there are any concerns about the medical management of the deceased. The second doctor is only able to complete the Cremation Form after seeing the body and discussing the death with the first doctor, and any person present at the time of death (The Shipman Inquiry, 2004). The properly completed medical certificate is checked by the Medical Referee at the chosen crematorium who gives final approval for cremation to occur.

Occasionally, circumstances occur in which the death must be reported to the coroner. The coroner will investigate deaths where:

- the deceased was not attended by a doctor during the last illness or the doctor treating the deceased had not seen the person either after death or within the 14 days before death;
- the death was violent or unnatural or occurred under suspicious circumstances;
- the cause of death is not known or is uncertain;
- the death occurred while the patient was undergoing an operation or did not recover from the anaesthetic;
- the death was caused by an industrial disease;
- the death occurred in prison or in police custody.

It is the duty of the registrar to report a death to a coroner but it is considered good practice for a doctor to do it directly as it reduces the distress to the family of the deceased and prevents delay (*R v Clark* [1702]; *R v Wiltshire Coroner ex p. Clegg* (1996)). Only some 3.4% of cases are reported to the coroner by the registrar (Home Office, 2003).

Once the doctor has reported the death to the coroner, a number of outcomes are possible. If the doctor is qualified to complete the medical certificate of cause of death certificate, that is the doctor attended the patient during his last illness, saw the patient within 14 days of his death or the body after death and is confident about the cause of death, then the matter may be discussed informally with the coroner and the certificate of cause of death completed and initialled on the back.

If the doctor is not qualified under the Births and Deaths Regulations 1987 to complete the certificate, the matter can still be discussed with the coroner who may decide that no action is necessary and he will issue a form 100A (no inquest or post-mortem necessary) to the Registrar.

If the cause of death is unknown, then the coroner is very likely to ask for a post-mortem. Where this confirms the cause of death as natural causes, it is open to the coroner to issue form B (100), no inquest following post-mortem, to the registrar: although the death was sudden, the cause is now known and does not warrant an inquest.

The coroner may decide after considering the post-mortem report and circumstances of the death to hold an inquest. If the cause of death is unnatural, the coroner will be obliged to hold an inquest. Until this has been completed, the patient's death will not be registered, although the coroner will be able to release the body for the funeral soon after the cause of death is known and issue an Order for Burial or Certificate for Cremation (Coroners Rules 1984, r.60). After the inquest the coroner will issue a Certificate after Inquest stating the cause of death to the registrar to allow the death to be registered.

An inquest can proceed with or without a jury. The coroner is obliged to have a jury present where:

- the death occurred in prison or in such a place or in such circumstances as to require an inquest under any other Act;
- the death occurred while the deceased was in police custody, or resulted from an injury caused by a police officer in the purported execution of his duty;
- the death was caused by an accident, poisoning or disease notice of which is required to be given under any Act to a government department, to any inspector or other officer of a government department or to an inspector appointed under the Health and Safety at Work Act 1974; or
- the death occurred in circumstances, the continuance or possible recurrence of which is prejudicial to the health or safety of the public or any section of the public.

A coroner's jury in England and Wales comprises between 7 and 11 people who are summonsed to serve in the normal way.

The inquest is a rare example of an inquisitorial trial where the aim is to establish the true circumstances of death. In an inquest it is the coroner who asks the majority of questions and who decides what evidence to allow. Where coroners are required to hold an inquest, they must inform the partner of the deceased or their nearest relative (Coroners Rules 1984, Rule 19; Coroners (Amendment) Rules 2005).

Following an inquest, the coroner will record the verdict as to how the deceased came to his/her death. A coroner may require action to be taken to prevent a recurrence and draw attention to these publicly and to any appropriate authority such as an NHS Trust.

PRACTICAL APPLICATION OF CONCEPT

Due to the nature of their work, nurses will undoubtedly encounter cases where patients die. Nurses have a vital role in assisting relatives through the process of verification of death, certification of death and registration of the death.

Some deaths will need to be reported to the coroner who is charged under the Coroners Act 1988 and its regulations to investigate the circumstances of death due to violent or unnatural causes or sudden deaths where the cause is unknown. Nurses must know when a death is likely to be reported to the coroner and be able to explain to relatives the likely course of events once such a report is submitted.

See also: concept of death; legal and ethical issues in palliative care; organ donation

FURTHER READING

Dorries, C. (2004) *Coroner's Courts: A Guide to Law and Practice*. Oxford: Oxford University Press.

Home Office (2004) *Reforming the Coroner and Death Certification Service: A Position Paper, Cm 6159*. London: TSO.

Ministry of Justice (2009) *Charter for Bereaved People who Come into Contact with a Reformed Coroner System*. London: TSO.

REFERENCES

Coroners (Amendment) Rules 2005 (SI 2005/420).

Coroners Rules 1984 (SI 1984/552).

Home Office (2003) *Death Certification and Investigation in England, Wales and Northern Ireland: The Report of a Fundamental Review (Cmd 5831)*. London: TSO.

The Shipman Inquiry (2004) *Fifth Report: Safeguarding Patients: Lessons from the Past – Proposals for the Future (Cm 6394)*. London: TSO.

CASES CITED

R v Clark [1702] 1 Salk 377
R v Wiltshire Coroner ex p. Clegg (1996) 161 JP 521

11 cultural issues
in palliative care

Shirley Firth

DEFINITION

Patients in palliative care may come from various religious groups, different ethnic groups, or be visibly different, yet thoroughly British. While there may be common characteristics and requirements of membership of any group, it is important not to stereotype patients, or have check lists, but to see each person as an individual who needs to feel valued and cared for, set into the context of a particular family who may want and need to be involved. Religious traditions and different health beliefs may also influence the way patients respond to treatment and the way they die; understanding these can improve care, sensitivity and awareness and help in the provision of an appropriate service. Ethnicity refers to shared descent and membership of a particular group although it is often associated with the country of origin. It is scientifically untenable to think in terms of 'race'. Culture has to do with the emotional and mental framework and guidelines which we inherit, yet which can also be acquired by newcomers. Religion refers both to membership of a particular faith community and also to the spiritual needs and practices of individuals (Helman, 1990).

cultural issues

49

KEY POINTS

Palliative care that takes account of culture requires knowledge and sensitivity in respect of the following:

- family structures and roles in relation to care and disclosure;
- referrals and access;
- communication;
- religious models of a good death;
- religious, spiritual and emotional needs;
- palliative care practice in the UK;
- bereavement;
- challenges for carers.

DISCUSSION

Many patients from the Indian Subcontinent and other Asian or African communities belong to extended families who expect to be involved in the care of the patients. In Southern Europe, too, decision-making is often in the hands of the senior members of the family, who may wish to control the giving of information about prognosis and disclosure. The professionalisation of care may make them feel disempowered, but failing in their duty to their loved ones may also have long-term repercussions.

Most people from minority communities want to die at home, although some Chinese and Africans prefer to die in hospital. However, there are low rates of referrals to palliative care services and hospices by some doctors who assume the community 'cares for their own'. Unless there has been an effective outreach programme, people may not know about available services and assume that hospices are where 'white people go to die' (Karim et al., 2000; Firth, 2001; Simmonds et al., 2001). The film, *Humara Safar*, is an excellent example of educating the Asian community. The 'Hospice at home' service may be difficult to provide because South Asians feel shame in asking for help if the illness, such as prostate cancer, is stigmatising. Thus there may be little support, even from relatives. For example, a carer such as a young Bangladeshi wife caring for a much older husband can be very lonely and have to depend on children who have to leave school to help (Firth, 2001). Africans, African Caribbeans and Irish men may not have family members in this country to provide care, and may suffer from the 'triple jeopardy' of poverty, illness and old age (Blakemore, 2000). There may be serious financial problems, and ignorance of available provisions.

Communication with different language speakers can often be difficult, and the use of children as interpreters is unfair on both parent and child, and violates the normal boundaries. Husbands or members of the community may tell both the wife and the medical staff what they think rather than what they want to say or know. Good interpreters can be hard to find among speakers of minority languages, but the ideal is to have properly trained patient advocates from the different ethnic communities, who can explain unfamiliar terminology, such as 'brain dead' and other medical terms, and also interpret what both doctor and patient are really saying (Firth, 2001; Gerrish et al., 2004).

Members of Black and Ethnic Minorities (BEMs) may be Christians, but those of other faiths need to have their beliefs and practices respected. There are already many booklets explaining their care needs, but here it needs to be emphasised that for many believers there is a concept of a good death, which may include:

- preparation for death;
- making a will (especially Muslims);
- saying goodbye;
- making gifts to charity;
- giving and asking forgiveness;
- arranging daughters' marriages;
- dying at home, although some Africans and Chinese may prefer hospital or hospice;
- the family being present;
- fasting for some;
- scripture readings/hymn singing;
- rituals, including penance;
- prayers or meditation to ensure the right state of mind at the point of death;
- Ganges water, tulsi, Amrit, Holy Water;
- facing Makkah (Muslims);
- death on floor for some Hindus and Sikhs;
- community support;
- the availability of a priest, imam, granthi or rabbi.

In the UK, none of these may be possible. There may be inadequate palliative care and few choices. The family may be fragmented or not available, or worse, excluded, so that the person dies alone, unable to follow the desired rituals, including ritual ablutions and last prayers. Yet for many it is immensely important both to the dying person and the survivors to die at peace, with the mind fixed on God. Religious functionaries may not be available or called. The family may not be informed about the prognosis or involved with discussion about care and disclosure may be made in a culturally inappropriate manner. Individuals from many countries may wish to die in their homeland and the practicalities need discussing sympathetically (Gardner 2002).

Nurses may feel inadequate in dealing with the religious and spiritual needs of patients of different traditions, especially if they do not feel confident of their own knowledge and understanding. They should never underestimate the value of just being a kind and loving presence, often without words, but with a gentle touch when appropriate (it may not be in the case of the opposite gender, but intuition can usually be trusted here). Even people of deep faith can feel fear and uncertainty. Having access to appropriate symbols and holy books can be comforting, and it is important to find other community members who can give help and comfort and perform last rites. If family members chant prior to death or weep loudly, then the tactful thing is to provide another room, where the considerable numbers and noise won't be disturbing (Gerrish et al., 1996).

For immigrants, the death may bring painful reminders of multiple losses, and a bad death which has not been in accordance with family and religious traditions causes more grief and anger. Loud crying may occur, or fainting. There may not be adequate bereavement support within their own communities (supposing they exist). Staff and bereavement counsellors need to familiarize themselves with different cultural expressions of emotion, and avoid stereotypical Western formulations (Firth, 2001).

Carers may be challenged by difference. Gunaratnam's concept of referential grounding recommends placing oneself in the shoes of the other person, and finding common aspects of experience (Gunaratnam et al., 1998). Cultural competence also means being self-aware, and examining one's own unconscious stereotyping and racism or prejudice (Leininger, 1996). Sharing with other staff and in-service training are invaluable. Reading articles about nursing patients from other cultures and finding out about different traditions will broaden understanding. Learning at least a few phrases in commonly spoken languages in the area where one works encourages trust and empathy. Visiting local temples, synagogues, mosques and gurdwaras also broadens one's experience, and establishes fruitful relationships. Ideally hospices should have outreach workers from minority ethnic communities, as well as patient advocates who speak the relevant languages (Firth, 2001; Simmonds et al., 2001).

PRACTICAL APPLICATION OF CONCEPT

Pushpa, a Hindu, has uterine cancer but has kept this secret out of shame. This has made treatment difficult. She brushes off in-patient treatment as 'just a check-up'. She refused chemotherapy as she had seen people's hair fall out and this would reveal her condition. Her husband works long shifts, demanding food whenever he gets home. She has two children, a boy of 8 and a daughter of 14, who miss school to help. As she deteriorates, the hospital wants to refer her to the palliative home care team, but she is ashamed to be seen to be asking for help. When she becomes weaker, the doctors want to refer her to a hospice for assessment and symptom management and for respite care, but she believes this is where white people dump their dying relatives. The hospice outreach worker, a Sikh, understands Pushpa's dilemma, and gently encourages her to talk openly with her family and relatives about her condition, offering to be present. She explains what the service can do. Despite their shock at the news, the husband and children are relieved by her assurances, as she is perceived as 'one of us'. They agree to visit the hospice with her. The hospice is so welcoming and understanding that they accept the offer of help.

See also: caring for the carers; communication; funerals; good death

FURTHER READING

Humara Safar (Our journey), made by SAPCAA (South Asian Palliative Care Awareness Arts Project), in Hindi, with English subtitles, aiming to raise awareness of palliative care among South Asian communities. Available on free loan from the Cancer Information Centre.

Oliviere, D. and Monroe, B. (2004) *Death, Dying and Social Difference*. Oxford: Oxford University Press.

Papadopoulos, I., Tilki, M. and Taylor, G. (1998) *Transcultural Care: A Guide for Health Care Professionals*. Salisbury: Quay Books.

REFERENCES

Blakemore, K. (2000) 'Health and social care in minority communities: an over-problematized issue?', *Health and Social Care in the Community*, 8(1): 22–30

Firth, S. (2001) *Wider Horizons: Care of the Dying in a Multicultural Community*. London: NCHSPCS.

Gardner, K. (2002) *Age, Narrative and Migration: The Life Course and Life Histories of Bangladeshi Elders in London*. London: Berg.

Gerrish, K., Chau, R., Sobowale, A. and Birks, E. (2004) 'Bridging the language barrier: the use of interpreters in primary care nursing', *Health and Social Care in the Community*, 12(5): 407–13.

Gerrish, K., Husband, C. and Mackenzie, J. (1996) *Nursing for a Multi-ethnic Society*. Buckingham: Open University Press.

Gunaratnam, Y., Bremner, I., Pollock, L. and Weir, C. (1998) 'Anti-discrimination, emotions and professional practice', *European Journal of Palliative Care*, 5(4): 122–4.

Helman, C. (1990) *Culture, Health and Illness*. Oxford: Butterworth-Heinemann Ltd.

Karim, K., Gailey, M. and Tunna, K. (2000) 'Non-white ethnicity and the provision of specialist palliative care services: factors affecting doctors' referral patterns', *Palliative Medicine*, 14: 471–8

Leininger, M. (1996) 'Response to Cooney article, "A comparative analysis of transcultural nursing and cultural safety"', *Nursing Praxis in New Zealand*, 22(2):13–15.

Simmonds, R., Sque, M., Goddard, G., Tullet, R. and Mount, J. (2001) *Improving Access to Palliative Care Services of Ethnic Minority Groups: A Report of a Study Funded by the Community Fund*. Crawley: St. Catherine's Hospice.

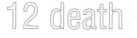

12 death

Jane Quigley

DEFINITION

Death is the cessation of life and a journey towards which individuals will make in their own unique way.

It's only when we truly know and understand that we have a limited time on earth – and that we have no way of knowing when our time is up, we will then begin to live each day to the fullest, as if it was the only one we had. (Kübler-Ross www.ekrfoundation.org)

How people die remains in the lasting memory of relatives, carers, health and social care staff and it is important that staff recognise their responsibility to provide the best possible care at the end of life (Department of Health, 2008: 64).

KEY POINTS

- Care at the end of life takes account of the person's dying trajectory.
- The way in which the dying and family members are living with dying.
- The dying person's last wishes.
- The final stage, the dying process.

DISCUSSION

The dying trajectory

The dying trajectory (or path) has two properties and takes place over time 'duration' and has 'shape', according to Dickenson and Johnson (2000). For some people, death happens suddenly from an accident, stroke or heart attack. For others, death comes after a long or protracted illness. The shape of a person's dying trajectory can be sudden; or a slow, constant deterioration; a stepwise decline, or a decline followed by a long plateau or remission, followed by fatal decline.

Dickenson and Johnson (2000: 218) discuss seven critical stages:

- Patient defined as dying.
- Staff and family make preparations for death which may include the dying person.
- Point at which nothing more can be done.
- Final descent – which can be weeks, days, or hours.
- The last hours.
- The death watch.
- Death itself.

Hallenbeck (2003) discusses the concept of a dying trajectory and refers to the change in health status over time as a patient approaches death. This concept has been helpful in understanding patterns of advanced illness and dying from different disease processes, all of which have implications for care needs, decision-making, and prognosis.

Cancer deaths often follow similar dying trajectories, as most patients with metastatic cancer remain quite functional until approximately five to six months

54

before their deaths. Their health then tends to slowly decline until the rate of decline accelerates rapidly two to three months before death. The hospice movement was developed primarily with this dying trajectory in mind. Prior to the rapid decline phase in the last few months or weeks, it may be hard to predict when patients with certain cancers will die, and the implications of this dying trajectory are that when the rapid decline phase begins, prediction of death in a matter of months or weeks is more certain than for most other diseases.

Long-term conditions such as congestive heart failure (CHF), chronic obstructive pulmonary disease (COPD), strokes, and many infirmities of advanced age follow a very different pattern. Acute exacerbations occur intermittently and tend to increase in frequency until patients often appear to be moving from chronic to acute ill health. People have trouble accepting the uncertainty in this trajectory and one of the most difficult tasks is helping patients and families through this.

The situation of sudden death is equally difficult as it is often those left behind who need the most immediate help and support. The characteristic of this trajectory is lack of preparation for dying. Usually those who die in this manner unless already very ill or of advanced age, will not have prepared for their death, and will not have had a chance to settle matters or say goodbye, and neither have those they leave behind.

Living with dying

It must be remembered that patients on any disease trajectory are likely to move between primary and secondary or tertiary care, and to be cared for by primary care teams, palliative care specialists and/or secondary care teams. Communication is vital ensuring that timely and relevant information is communicated to all other professionals involved, particularly at times of transition from one care setting to another.

As health professionals we are able to influence a family's capacity to cope with death and dying, making the final hours as peaceful as possible. At the end, death may occur rapidly and it is essential that families are involved, if they wish to be, in order to gain their acceptance and understanding. Patients and relatives need information about the illness itself and what to watch for if they are to carry the ongoing responsibility for care. They need factual information to plan their own lives and in order to be prepared. This may include information on the likely course of the illness, financial benefits and entitlements, compassionate leave, and what to do when someone dies.

When a patient is admitted to hospital or a care home, families should not feel excluded and be allowed to help with care. Equally, caring for a person at home may leave relatives overwhelmed and even carers who are health professionals may need the help and support of services in the community. However, at times, professionals may not know what to do, or may not have the resources available to ensure maximum comfort for the patient and support for relatives. As a result, many people experience unnecessary physical, psychological and spiritual suffering and many do not live out their final days in the way they would have chosen. It can also influence the way family and friends cope during the dying process and during bereavement (Department of Health, 2008).

Patient and family experiences of death and dying are thought to be affected by the lack of familiarity with such concepts and events as a result of modern society and the way we live.

> Different generations are less likely to live together, and deaths are more likely to happen outwith the family home than in the past. The resulting cultural resistance to acknowledging the reality of death and dying as an inevitable and integral parts of life and reluctance to discuss these, particularly in the context of a health service focussed on 'cure' rather than 'care', can contribute to poor communication and planning of end of life care. (The Scottish Government, 2008: 4).

Talking about the death of someone close may be difficult, yet talking and recalling memories and sharing feelings may be important in the grief process. When death has been protracted, the family may also have suffered a prolonged period of stress in which they felt unable to undertake normal activities, having faced a period focused on the person who was dying, to the detriment of themselves and others.

Last wishes

When faced with the knowledge that they are entering the final stages of their lives, some patients may choose to think about how they would prefer to die. Some will have strong opinions and feel the need to secure promises from family members that their wishes will be honoured, even if they get to a stage when they are unable to speak for themselves. Listening to a terminally ill patient and offering reassurance that they are being understood can provide them with a great sense of comfort. Whether they wish to fight until the very last moments or come to a point of wanting to be at home, without any medical intervention, knowing that their choices will be respected, is important.

'So many aspects of the dying process are out of the control of those involved. Illness takes its own course and death comes when it wishes, but there are things that can be done to help patients and their loved ones to individualise the experience as much as possible' (Terminal Illness.co.uk). This is addressed in the *End of Life Care Strategy* (Department of Health, 2008) with a focus on discussing such issues with patients and their families.

The dying process

Personal experience, fear, cultural issues, professional and individual concerns all affect the way we deal with patients facing death. Identifying that a person is dying is difficult, even for experienced professionals, but various signs will suggest that a person may be in the last days or hours of life. They may become more withdrawn and slip in and out of consciousness, and those caring for them should recognise a person is dying and take appropriate action to support both the patient and the relative.

Signs and symptoms of imminent death may be:

- lowered body temperature – cold hands and extremities;
- decreased intake of fluids;
- skin colour changes as circulation slows down; lips and nail beds may have blue tinge;
- sunken cheeks, relaxation of facial muscles;
- rattles in chest – breathing may be more laboured;
- Cheyne-Stokes respirations;
- the pulse becomes irregular and may slow down or speed up, blood pressure lowers;
- restlessness or confusion;
- sweating. (adapted from Woodhouse, 2005)

Signs of approaching death may vary as it will be affected by the illness and treatment. Breathing may become more irregular and often slower. Cheyne-Stokes breathing, rapid breathing followed by periods of no breathing, may occur. Congestion in the airway can increase, causing 'noisy' breathing which may be distressing for relatives, and it should be explained it is not an indication of pain or suffering. Hands and feet may become blotchy and mottled as circulation slows down. Patients may be unresponsive and have their eyes open but not seeing their surroundings which again may distress relatives. It is not unusual for dying persons to experience sensory changes. Sometimes a patient may appear confused about a sound or object in the room. They might hear a noise and think someone is crying or think they see someone in the room. They may hear things you cannot hear, see things that you cannot see, or feel things that you are unable to touch or feel and relatives may need reassurance if this happens.

It is widely believed that hearing is the last sense to go so it is important that relatives are encouraged to talk and say the things they need to say. Coma or a state of deep unconsciousness may occur, however, even in this state patients may still hear though they may not respond. Eventually, breathing will cease and the heart stops and at this point death has occurred.

CONCLUSION

Health and social care professionals are privileged to be able to support patients and relatives helping them to recognise and prepare for death. They may need to know that they should just be themselves and relate to the person as they always did, be ready to listen to them and be aware of what they don't say as much as what they do, and that what often matters most to a person who is dying is simply taking time to hold a hand, give support and just be there.

PRACTICAL APPLICATION OF CONCEPT

Keith's story – adapted from his wife's words – (Department of Health, 2008: 25). Following surgery to remove an intestinal tumour, Keith developed an abscess that perforated, necessitating him being ventilated and nursed on an intensive care unit. During this time his wife stayed with him constantly, sometimes sleeping in the hospital waiting room as there was nowhere else for her to stay.

Keith regained consciousness and when his condition stabilised he was moved back to a general ward. His wife was told that the bowel cancer had not spread and staff felt that he could return home within five days. However, Keith stopped eating and two days later his pain had increased significantly. His wife described spending hours one evening trying to speak to random doctors and nurses about his condition, before eventually returning home. The following day she phoned and was told that Keith had gone back to intensive care and was ventilated. Staff did not tell her that she could return to the hospital immediately and so she didn't, as previously she had been 'told off' for sleeping in the hospital waiting room.

Although not directly told, Keith's wife suspected that his life was limited. As a result she was unsure about contacting her four children. She also struggled with the decision about informing Keith's priest, as she did not want to alarm her husband but at the same time she knew he would wish to see a priest. She also felt upset and cheated that she had not been able to say goodbye to her husband before he was re-ventilated.

Keith's children were distressed to see their father connected to a ventilator and unable to speak. Keith's wife recalls the hospital staff saying that they would not resuscitate Keith if his heart stopped. However, she was not involved in any of these decisions and two days later Keith was still being given invasive treatments. Looking back, Keith's wife felt that had she been involved in decisions about his care she would have requested that unnecessary treatments should have stopped.

After a period, the hospital staff informed her that they had stopped giving Keith drugs, but they did not explain what would happen to Keith as a result. When she asked how she would know he had died, she was told to 'watch the equipment, when it reaches zero he will have died'. So, with her children, she watched until Keith died.

How people die remains in the memory of those who live on. (Saunders, 1989)

See also: *caring for the carers; concept of death*

FURTHER READING

Department of Health (2008) *End of Life Care Strategy – Promoting High Quality Care for All Adults at the End of Life*. London: Department of Health. Available at:

key concepts in palliative care

www.dh.gov.uk/en/Publicationsandstatistics/Publications/PublicationsPolicy AndGuidance/
DH_086277 accessed 18 June 2009.
Liverpool Care Pathway for the Dying Patient (LCP) website. www.mcpcil.org.uk/liver-
pool_care_pathway accessed 18 June 2009.

REFERENCES

Department of Health (2008) *End of Life Care Strategy – Promoting High Quality Care for
All Adults at the End of Life*. London: DH.
Dickenson, D. and Johnson, M. (2000) *Death, Dying and Bereavement*. Milton Keynes: The
Open University Press.
Hallenbeck, J. (2003) *Palliative Care Perspectives*. Oxford: Oxford University Press.
Kübler-Ross, E. www.ekrfoundation.org accessed 18 June 2009.
Saunders, C. (1989) 'Pain and impending death', in P.D. Wall and R. Melzak (eds), *Textbook
of Pain*, 2nd edn. Edinburgh: Churchill Livingstone, pp. 624–31.
The Scottish Government (2008) *Living and Dying Well: A National Action Plan for Palliative
and End of Life Care in Scotland*. Edinburgh: The Scottish Government.
Terminal Illness.co.uk. www.terminalillness.co.uk/respecting-a-patients-wishes.html
accessed 18 June 2009.
Woodhouse, J. (2005) 'A personal reflection on sitting at the bedside of a dying loved one:
the final hours of life', *International Journal of Palliative Nursing*, 11(1): 28–32.

13 environment of care: palliative care within the acute hospital care ward

John Costello

DEFINITION

The context in which palliative care is provided is an important determinant
in the end of life experience. The majority of people who die in the UK each

year do so in hospital (Department of Health, 2008). This means that by and large a significant number of patients receive palliative care in this context at the end of life. This has implications for influencing decisions about the preferred place of care documentation (Department of Health, 2004) currently enabling patients to state preferences and to become involved in shaping their end of life care.

The aim of this chapter is to consider some of the challenges to providing effective palliative care in this context as well as some of the advantages of enabling hospital patients to experience a good death. The chapter begins by considering the nature of the curative approach which is embedded in the acute care context as well as the implications this has for providing optimal palliative care experiences for adult patients and their families. The argument is made that for patients and families to receive optimal palliative care, it is necessary to be open and honest about the diagnosis and prognosis and therefore discuss their impending death in order to achieve, what for them, is a good death. The chapter concludes by focusing on the practical application, based on an assessment of the patient's preferred place of care at the end of life.

KEY POINTS

- There are differences of ideologies in the environment of care: cure versus care.
- Disclosing information about the patient's prognosis is necessary for a 'good death'.
- Contemporary palliative care includes supportive care for the family.

DISCUSSION

Acute care in hospital: cure versus care

The majority of people in the UK die in hospital despite research indicating that their preferred place of care is at home (Department of Health, 2008). End of life care in acute hospital settings has many challenges, not least of which is the need to enable the patient and family to experience a good death (Costello, 2006). There is a wealth of research indicating that nurses and doctors in hospitals operate on the basis of the medical model and that despite very significant changes in the last decade, end of life care in hospitals remains very medicalised (Clark, 2002). Hospitals were originally designed to cure the sick and were never devised as ideal places in which to die. Today there are numerous challenges such as ward routines, power struggles between staff groups and the development of a business culture. The latter places pressure on staff to discharge patients as quickly as possible and to prevent others from becoming what is referred to as *bed blockers*.

The emphasis on much contemporary hospital care is placed on throughput, output and turnover. This leaves little room for focusing on the needs of the patient, their wishes and preferences, and what constitutes dying well. Good death situations involve the patients and their family being involved in decision-making at the end of life, as well as experiencing death with dignity and peace. These become difficult when the patient is cared for in a bay of other patients, who may be recovering from surgery or admitted for investigations. Notwithstanding these difficulties, nurses and others can, and do, rise to the challenge of enabling patients and families to experience death with dignity in acute hospital settings. Good deaths take place in hospital because nurses apply sensitive and compassionate care. This is achieved by developing therapeutic relationships with patients and by getting to know and addressing the needs of family members at the end of life (Hopkinson et al., 2003). However, discussing death and planning end of life care involves hospital staff in disclosing the diagnosis, (often called breaking bad news), that can, and does, involve complex negotiation with the patient and family. Without knowing the truth about the diagnosis and having a realistic idea of the future, it is difficult for hospital staff to engage the patient and family in advance end of life care planning.

Disclosing information: talking about death and dying

The phenomenon of dying in hospital is cloaked in secrecy. Nurses' attempts to conceal death from patients by closing curtains and not disclosing information about individual deaths reflect discomfort about what is, in some settings, a regular event. Research findings suggest that nurses want patients to die without distress, including distress to themselves and others in the settings in which they work (Costello, 2006). Nurses often preferred 'medicalised deaths' which optimised control, compared with more natural deaths that were unpredictable and sometimes prolonged. A good death needs to include a degree of social control, with the patient in a position in which they are 'ready to die'. This type of preparation begins with diagnosis and requires a high level of communication between nurses, patients and multiprofessional groups. It also requires nurses to challenge custom and cultural practices that seek to deny death as a social reality and demonstrate a lack of dignity about death itself. In particular, it is not the death event itself that is important, but the process of dying and the extent to which patient and family expectations are met through effective and sensitive communication. Disclosure of information about a patient's death can begin by assessing what the patient knows about their illness when *bad news* is broken. Good practice dictates that those breaking bad news elicit the patient and family concerns and try to give an open and honest account of the prognosis (Kalber, 2009). From this point, nurses are often required to monitor a patient's progress and in many cases an Integrated Care Pathway (ICP) is used to identify changes and variance in the patient's physical and psychological condition (Ellershaw and Wilkinson, 2003).

The role of the nurse in providing optimal palliative care at the end of life is to engage with the patient and family and find out what their concerns are and how these may be addressed. This will obviously include assessment of pain and other symptoms and providing means of alleviating these symptoms. At the same time, it is important to focus on psychological, social and spiritual issues. To do this, it is useful to develop a relationship based on trust, compassion and empathy (Griffiths, 2008). Such relationships focus on the practitioner, who engages with the family by informing, identifying and advocating, based on a clear understanding of the patient's wishes. Central to enabling the patient and family to experience a good death is the notion of finding out their perceptions about end of life care and their preferred place of care. The Preferred Place of Care (redesignated Preferred Priorities of Care [PPC], Department of Health, 2008) documentation is designed to enable patients to exercise choice and for practitioners to act in accordance with the important ethical principle of patient autonomy to elicit patient needs. In itself, the documentation can be used as a strategy to develop dialogue about dying and importantly, focus on the patient's wishes rather than the needs of the hospital and its staff. Rather than use euphemisms to talk about death, the document is a means of discussing sensitive issues such as 'who will care for me?' and 'how will my symptoms be controlled?'. By working collaboratively to achieve patient outcomes for care palliative care teams, together with other hospital disciplines, can offer patients choice and enable the rhetoric of a good death to become a reality.

Supportive care

Contemporary palliative care includes meeting the social, psychological and spiritual care concerns of the patient and the family and is often referred to as holistic care. Supportive care, however, focuses attention on the needs of the family members as often, it is those closest to the patients who share the distress of impending loss. In this respect, healthcare practitioners have an obligation to enable the end of life to be as peaceful as possible and for every patient to die well. The notion of a good death is highlighted by a number of authors (Hopkinson et al., 2003; Vig & Pearlman, 2004; Costello, 2006), and others who point up the need for effective supportive care to be provided by all practitioners especially at the end of life in order to enable family members to experience a good death (Thompson-Hill et al., 2009). The following vignette taken from a clinical practice scenario highlights this issue.

PRACTICAL APPLICATION OF THE CONCEPT

Harry was a 66-year-old widower with cancer of the pancreas who had a only a few weeks to live. His son Mark and daughter-in-law Carole felt devastated, especially as his wife had died of cancer less than a year ago. Jason, the nurse who admitted Harry, was aware of the situation and arranged for Mark and

Carole to see the consultant privately to discuss end of life issues as Mark found it very difficult to have conversations about death with his father. Mark agreed to talk to Harry about where he would like to die using the Preferred Place of Care guidance. Harry wanted to die at home but felt that he would be a burden to his son if this was to happen. A care package was arranged and the rapid discharge team became involved. Jason arranged for the Hospital Macmillan nurse to liaise with her community partner and together they spoke to Harry and his son. Harry was discharged home five days later with district nurses and Macmillan support. His son and daughter-in-law took time off work and together they managed to care for Harry until he died peacefully at home three weeks later.

Harry's story is slightly atypical although it embraces the notion of multi-professional teamwork. It demonstrates that with the motivation and desire to apply the principles of supportive and palliative care, patients, while in hospital, can achieve their preferred place of care at the end of life, and experience a good death.

See also: caring for the carers; communication; good death, multi-disciplinary teams

FURTHER READING

Costello, J. (2004) *Nursing the Dying Patient: Caring in Different Contexts.* London: Palgrave.
Lugton, J. and Kindlen, M. (2000) *Palliative Care: The Nursing Role.* London: Churchill Livingstone.

REFERENCES

Clark, D. (2002) 'Between hope and acceptance: the medicalisation of dying', *British Medical Journal*, 324: 905–7.
Costello, J. (2006) 'Dying well: nurses' experiences of good and bad deaths in hospital', *Journal of Advanced Nursing*, 54(5): 1–8.
Department of Health (2004) *Preferred Place of Care.* London: DH.
Department of Health (2008) *The End of Life Care Strategy: Promoting High Quality of Care for All Adults at the End of Life.* London: DH.
Ellershaw, J. and Wilkinson, S. (2003) *Care of the Dying: A Pathway to Excellence.* Oxford: Oxford University Press.
Griffiths, P. (2008) 'The art of losing…? A response to the question "is caring a lost art?"', *International Journal of Nursing Studies*, 45: 329–32.
Hopkinson, J.B., Hallett, C.E. and Luker, K.A. (2003) 'Caring for dying people in hospital', *Journal of Advanced Nursing*, 44(5): 525–33.
Kalber, B. (2009) 'Breaking bad news – whose responsibility is it?', *European Journal of Cancer Care*, 18(4): 330.
Thompson-Hill, J., Hookey, C., Salt, E. and O'Neill, T. (2009) 'The Supportive Care Plan: a tool to improve communication in end of life care', *International Journal of Palliative Nursing*, 15(5): 250–5.
Vig, E.K. and Pearlman, R.A. (2004) 'Good and bad dying from the perspective of terminally ill men', *Archive of Internal Medicine*, 164(9): 977–81.

environment of care

14 finance issues and the organisation of palliative care

Peter Hartland

DEFINITION

Palliative care services are delivered at local community level within a framework guided by national policy and regulation, through a variety of service providers accessing a number of sources of funding. The distributed and differing nature of services makes both access to and extent of palliative care variable across regions.

KEY POINTS

Finance issues in respect of organisation of palliative care take account of the following:

- delivery mechanisms and providers;
- national guidance;
- regulation;
- education and research;
- funding;
- expenditure profiles and standard costs;
- future trends.

DISCUSSION

Although all clinicians will be familiar with some general palliative care principles and techniques, the application of specialist palliative care – most often in an End of Life (EOL) setting – is, as the name suggests, a highly specialised and intensive process. These specialist services are normally focused in a number of different service providers within each Primary Care Trust (PCT) area or region, and in some cases individual providers deliver services across a number of PCT areas. Examples of providers might be hospices, specialist centres at acute hospitals, or other charitable organisations supported by healthcare-related charities. In addition, many GP practices will receive education in specialist palliative care to enable them to assist in the correct treatment routes for patients.

Although still associated with the treatment of cancer, specialist palliative care is now being accessed more widely by patients suffering from other life-limiting conditions, for example, motor-neurone disease. In many cases patients receive palliative treatment outside of the 'traditional' in-patient setting and are now more frequently discharged to spend their last precious days at home, supported by specialist services where available.

Delivery mechanisms and providers

Hospices are still the major provider of in-patient resources for specialist palliative care. Hospices are funded through a combination of charitable income and NHS resourcing, varying from institution to institution, with no overall national guidance. 'Help the Hospices' provides a national voice for the hospice movement, acting as a conduit to government as well as resource base for training, support, guidance and collective activity. Hospices have developed significantly from the widely held perception of an in-patient ward; many now provide community services (often with an outreach to a patient base many times that delivered at the hospice site), as well as day centres for those patients who do not require intensive treatment, and often providing education resources (or a focal point) for palliative care learning, as well as extensive social and pastoral care and bereavement support. As they focus more on excellence in delivery of specialist palliative care, there is a reducing focus on pure 'respite care' which was often a feature of the service. Hospices continue to develop ground-breaking environments for patients and carers – both physical design and activity based, and the mixture of both NHS-based and locally employed clinicians, together with the charitable dynamic with extensive volunteer support, make for a unique service.

Specialist Units are a feature of larger hospitals and although these tend to provide less bed space than hospices their location within the acute setting makes them particularly flexible and highly utilised. The services provide a less extensive package of individual care than is possible at hospices, but they have access to the same level of specialised clinical support. Many consultants and doctors share their time between hospices and NHS providers as part of collective service support across an area.

National guidance – the NHS provides guidance on the delivery of key services, for example, the national *End of Life Care Strategy* (Department of Health, 2008a), published in July 2008, was informed and shaped by the work on end of life care undertaken by strategic health authorities for the NHS Next Stage Review (Department of Health, 2008b), known by many as 'The Darzi Report'. This strategy, and other directional guidance, inform local strategy and influence local delivery via the strategic health authorities and the PCTs (who commission services). There remain inconsistencies in commissioning, provision and funding as a result of local interpretation and prioritisation.

Regulation – all providers are regulated by the Care Quality Commission, the national agency tasked with ensuring proper standards of care delivery for healthcare providers and care homes. Regulation is undertaken through assessments, inspections and audits. In addition, hospices and other charitable providers are subject to the requirements of the Charity Commission, which imposes obligations over legal structure, governance, scope of activities, risk management, and financial viability and probity.

Education and research – strategic health authorities take a lead in ensuring that specialist palliative care training is available to clinicians, and often provide resources via hospices to enable modules to be available for undergraduate and postgraduate education. Providers often work in liaison with local university hospitals to coordinate education and research in specialist palliative care.

Funding – while service provision delivered within NHS trusts is directly funded through contracts with local PCTs, the hospice model is very different and highly variable. As independent bodies, hospices will hold a voluntary body/third sector contractor agreement with their PCT. This will specify a level of services to be provided, but will have a financial component that would normally only cover a percentage of the costs of the services, with the balance coming from the hospice's own charitable fundraising, investment income or endowed funds. The 'PCT percentage' varies from hospice to hospice (sometimes dependent on service levels, sometimes on historical funding levels), and is most normally in the range of 30–40% of total hospice expenditure. In children's hospices, where fundraising potential is seen as higher, this might be as low as 10% or less. Hospices' ability to raise their own funds is localised and variable; some have 'commercial' interests through the operation of 'second-hand' retail shop networks, some have their own lotteries, but all will have a highly community focused fundraising operation seeking donations, legacy support, event and activity income. For hospices there is increasing difficulty in competing with national charities (for a multitude of good causes) with significant marketing budgets. The recent recession has had a significant impact on hospices' fundraised income, as well as that generated from investments. In addition to 'monetary contributions', hospices rely on the donation of time from volunteers who often provide as much as 10% of the necessary 'human resource support' free of charge.

Expenditure profiles and standard costs – hospice costs are largely staff based – specialist palliative care is a highly intensive process; it is not a homogenous service, with every patient (especially those at end of life) requiring individualised care and support, and in many cases with secondary, tertiary and further conditions (both of a physical and mental nature). As a result, a 'tariff' approach to end of life specialist palliative care has not been achieved, and 'standard costs' for treatment do not exist. Most hospices would see at least 75% of their cost base being employee-based, showing the high level of human interaction required. This leads to financial difficulties where NHS-based wage inflation is not matched by PCT funding increases on an annual basis, putting extreme pressure on the fundraising activities of the organisation.

Future trends – the End-of-Life Care Strategy (Department of Health, 2008a) provides a number of challenges to specialist palliative care provision, not least in the desire to give patients a choice to receive support so that they can choose to remain at home. This poses questions over the need for, and extent of, specialist palliative care beds; it also gives rise to funding issues given the difficulty in quantifying the cost of individualised care at home and how this could be arranged. The Strategy earmarks specific monies funding streams to assist in the processes it advocates, but the exact cascade of those funds through the varying layers of the strategic and commissioning bodies to the actual providers is yet to be demonstrated.

PRACTICAL APPLICATION OF THE CONCEPT

St Luke's Hospice in Sheffield opened in 1971 following the pioneering work of its Founder, Professor Eric Wilkes. The Hospice now provides a 30-bedded inpatient centre, a day centre capable of supporting 20 patients per day, a community team supporting in excess of 300 patients at any time, as well as a full range of patient and carer wellbeing, social, pastoral and bereavement service – and with an education centre. The Hospice receives approximately 31% of its recurrent funding from its PCT. This recurrent funding percentage has reduced steadily over a number of years, as the annual inflation increase has lagged behind the increases seen in the real cost base – largely driven by the need to compete with NHS providers to recruit and retain staff, as well as to adhere to ever stricter and more prescriptive regulation. As a consequence, St Luke's needs to increase its fundraising income by around £200,000 each year, just to stand still. That represents an *extra* 40p from every woman, man and child in the city every year; or about 15% growth in fundraising income year-on-year.

See also: *organisational management of palliative care*

FURTHER READING

Tebbit, P. (2007) *Focus on Commissioning – End of Life Care: A Commissioning Perspective.* London: National Council for Palliative Care.

REFERENCES

Department of Health (2008a) *End of Life Care Strategy: Promoting High Quality Care for All Adults at the End of Life.* London: Department of Health.

Department of Health (2008b) *High Quality Care for All: NHS Next Stage Review Final Report* (summary letter by Lord Darzi). London: Department of Health.

finance issues

15 financial aspects for patients and carers

Jan Woodhouse

DEFINITION

Financial concerns fall into the category of 'social pain' when considering the concept of total pain that patients with palliative care needs experience. Knowledge of some of the issues, and how to resolve them, will therefore be useful for any health care practitioner.

KEY POINTS

- Illness brings a financial burden with it.
- There are a range of financial concerns, some of which may have a major impact on the patient and family.
- There are key times when financial advice could be offered.
- There are a variety of benefits available to patients with palliative care needs, in the UK.
- Specialists, such as benefit advisors and social workers, should be part of the multi-disciplinary team.

DISCUSSION

When illness appears, it may also usher in money shortages reducing those days of joy to days of despair. Perusing the literature on financial issues for patients and carers it appears that financial concerns emerge when participants in studies are asked about factors that have impacted on end-of-life experiences (Steinhauser et al., 2004; Scannell-Desch, 2005). This shows that financial concerns may be in the minds of the patients and carers but may not form the topic of conversation with healthcare professionals, for whom illness and disease is the focus of attention. However, if the healthcare professionals are trying to address patients' anxieties and support them and their carers, then perhaps the knowledge of what exactly might be affecting them may be useful.

Some specific financial concerns have been identified (Aranda and Peerson, 2001; Scannell-Desch, 2005; Knops et al., 2005; Steele and Davies, 2006) as:

- Having to give up work.
- Living on social security.
- Watching savings dwindle away.
- Borrowing against assets (life insurance, house).
- Selling assets.
- Paying the mortgage, rent and debts.
- Paying utility bills (which may be higher than normal, in order to keep the patient warm).
- Paying for carers and respite care.
- Paying for equipment.
- Paying for supportive services, such as counselling.
- Paying for special foods or diets.
- Transportation and parking costs.
- Paying for treats for the patient (or siblings, in the case of ill children).
- Not paying comprehensive health insurance or taking out life insurance.
- Funeral expenses.

Downsizing or moving house (and the contingent costs), both pre- and post-bereavement, were also noted in the studies by Scannell-Desch (2005) and Steele and Davies (2006).

It is interesting to note that most of the studies that go into depth about finance are American, Canadian or Australian and it may be that this is a consequence of how healthcare is paid for by the individual in those countries. In the UK, where the NHS is free at the point of delivery, these issues are perhaps not as stark. Never-the-less, looking at the above list, there is universality in respect of illness and its impact on finances. The Macmillan Cancer care organisation has taken great strides in raising the awareness of the financial aspects of illness and they provide information on a breadth of topics (Macmillan Cancer Support, 2009). Their website (Macmillan Learn Zone, 2008) notes that it is important that patients and carers take financial advice early, in order to save time and money. The time in the patient's journey when such advice might be needed, are:

- at time of diagnosis;
- undergoing treatment;
- changes in personal circumstances;
- when discharged from hospital;
- changes in medical condition;
- when other more general aspects arise, such as debts and housing problems.

The Department of Health (2004) recognises that illness brings a financial burden and has a booklet *Help with Health Costs* that is available for patients and carers to read. Financial help, for those on a low income, can be obtained through the NHS for the cost of prescriptions, dental care, glasses and sight tests, wigs, and travel costs to a hospital. However, this seems a limited list compared to what is actually needed. Where carers are needed or the patient's condition involves a degree of disability, then the Department of Work and Pensions has information on:

- Disability allowance;
- Attendance allowance;
- Carers allowance.

When the patient is recognised to be in the palliative care stage, defined as their death is expected within 6 months, then special rules apply. The special rules mean that there is no qualifying time required to receiving the allowance, unlike others, who have not reached a palliative care stage, who are applying for the allowance and have to demonstrate an ongoing need. Initiation of the special rules requires a GP or specialist to complete a form known as DS 1500, which requires details of the patient's condition and the form is then submitted along with the patient's claim form (Patient UK, 2009). In an audit carried out by Levy and Payne (2006: 327), the most frequent claims were for: 'income support, disability living allowance, council tax benefit, housing benefit, carers allowance, attendance allowance and incapacity benefit'.

In terms of equipment needs, items such as communication aids (charts, electronic voice devices, adapted computers) and walking aids (walking sticks, zimmers, etc.) are available at a reduced cost. Occupational therapists are usually aware of the range of equipment that is available and local schemes that exist. Low-income patients may be able to gain funds from a Community Care Grant in order to buy items such as clothing, bedding, washing machine, carpeting and fans. A Macmillan Grant may also provide for such items but Macmillan Cancer Care also considers aspects that improve the quality of life such as specialised furniture, fuel and heating bills, and holiday breaks (Macmillan Cancer Support, 2008).

So who does the patient or the carer turn to if they need financial advice? If they have access to the Internet, then government and charitable organisations, such as those mentioned above plus others such as Age Concern, Carers UK and the British Heart Foundation, also provide information on the topic. However, the jargon, the forms, and the time it takes to complete them can be off-putting for many individuals. Advice can be sought on the telephone and there exists the following:

- *Benefits Enquiry Line (BEL)*, whose number changes depending on which part of the UK you live in.
- *Carers Allowance Unit*, again the number changes depending on location.
- *Macmillan benefits advisor* (an interactive map on their website will find the nearest one to your location) – plus they also operate an e-mail question service.
- *Age Concern Information Line*, which operates from 8 am–7 pm.

For those who prefer a face-to-face encounter, then it is possible to discuss such issues with a local social worker, Macmillan specialist nurse or the Citizen Advice Bureau personnel. The latter agency, Levy and Payne (2006) note, may not have the specialist knowledge that the patient with palliative care needs demands. They go on to comment that only a few hospices have access to specialist welfare benefits advisors, meaning that there is a paucity of advisory help available to patients and carers. Macmillan specialist nurses do have an awareness of the benefits and the eligibility for claiming them. However, for those patients who do not have a cancer diagnosis, there appears to be poor support in respect of financial advice.

Patients with palliative care needs are often focused on the illness and the effects of the illness can impair concentration and the ability to read (Levy and Payne, 2006), so that filling out forms may become increasingly difficult. It may fall upon healthcare workers, and these are usually nurses, to help and assist the patient, or their carers, at this time. Admission or assessment documentation can often identify where financial advice is required but, as Levy and Payne (2006) note, these aspects can also be overlooked. Occasionally the financial situation of the patient is so severe, e.g. homelessness, or mounting debts, that it can involve a considerable workload for a social worker. A complex case may involve over a 100 telephone calls, the writing of numerous letters, and perusal of documents received from benefits agencies. It can be an arduous process for all concerned. However, if the financial burden is somehow alleviated at this difficult time, it may help in achieving a 'good death' for the patient and reduce the impact of bereavement for the carers. There is, then, a case to be made to include financial advisors to be available in all settings where palliative care is given, as a matter of course rather than waiting for the topic to crop up in conversation.

PRACTICAL APPLICATION OF THE CONCEPT

Henry was 60, lived alone and had a brain tumour. His brother, who had also had cancer, was aware of the benefits that were available to Henry. Together they filled out the necessary forms and organised some home care. An adjustable bed was purchased and grab rails were fitted in the shower. However, Henry was reluctant to accept help from the available services, relying on friends instead. The friends bought items such as food, cooking utensils and additional bedding when Henry's condition deteriorated. Even when he was admitted to hospital for the final weeks of his life, they continued to bring in treats that they knew Henry would like.

See also: funerals; good death; resources and information

FURTHER READING

Department of Work and Pensions website (www.dwp.gov.uk)
Macmillan Cancer Support organisation website (www.macmillan.org.uk)

REFERENCES

Aranda, S., and Peerson, A. (2001) 'Caregiving in advanced cancer: lay decision making', *Journal of Palliative Care*, 17(4): 270–6.

Department of Health (2004) *Help with Health Costs*. London: DH.

Knops, K.M., Srinivasan, M. and Meyers, F.J. (2005) 'Patient desires: a model for assessment of patient preferences for care of severe or terminal illness', *Palliative and Supportive Care*, 3: 289–99.

Levy, J. and Payne, M. (2006) 'Welfare rights advocacy in a specialist health and social care setting: a service audit', *British Journal of Social Work*, 36: 323–31.

Macmillan Cancer Support (2008) Macmillan Learn Zone: benefits awareness. Available at: http://learnzone.macmillan.org.uk/course/view.php?id=4, accessed 24 November 2008.

Macmillan Cancer Support (2009) Financial issues. Available at: www.macmillan.org.uk/Cancerinformation/Livingwithandaftercancer/Financialissues/Financialissues.aspx, accessed 14 October 2009.

Patient UK (2009) Benefits for the terminally ill. Available at: www.patient.co.uk/health/Benefits-for-the-Terminally-Ill.htm, accessed 14 October 2009.

Scannell-Desch, E.A. (2005) 'Pre-bereavement and post-bereavement struggles and triumphs of midlife widows', *Journal of Hospice and Palliative Nursing*, 7(1): 15–22.

Steinhauser, K.E., Clipp, E.C., Bosworh, H.B., McNeilly, M., Christakis, N.A., Voils, C.I. and Tulsky, J.A. (2004) 'Measuring quality of life at the end of life: validation of the QUAL-E', *Palliative and Supportive Care*, 2: 3–14.

Steele, R. and Davies, B. (2006) 'Impact on parents when a child has a progressive, life-threatening illness', *International Journal of Palliative Nursing*, 12(12): 576–85.

16 funerals

Jan Woodhouse

DEFINITION

The notion of discussing funerals in terms of palliative care may be seen as insensitive, perhaps somewhat pre-emptive, after all the patient hasn't yet died. However, thinking about one's own funeral is probably something we all engage in from time to time, from the moment we have an understanding of death and the ensuing disposal of a body.

A funeral, as defined by the *Compact Oxford English Dictionary*, is 'a ceremony in which a dead person is buried or cremated' (www.askoxford.com 2009). The timing of the ceremony can vary, depending on the religion of the deceased, the circumstances of the death, or the last wishes of the deceased or their family. Staff working in palliative care should have an awareness of these aspects.

KEY POINTS

- Healthcare professionals are key members in certifying the death and starting the funeral process.
- Funeral arrangements alter according to the religious practices of the patient.
- Patients and their family may be concerned about the costs of funeral.
- Children are now more likely to attend funerals, as societal attitudes change.

DISCUSSION

Healthcare professionals, working with patients who have palliative care needs, may get drawn into conversations, either with the patients or with the relatives, about the last hours of life and the funeral arrangements post-death. In addition, staff have responsibilities in respect of certifying the death and the laying the body out before it is collected by a funeral director. As such, it is a difficult time for all concerned, as information about religious observance, last wishes and statutory legislation have to be obtained and merged in order to address the care of the deceased.

The sociologist Tony Walters, who writes extensively on death and dying, once said at a conference that 'you can't get through death without the paper-work', and he is right. Staff need to be stringent in ensuring that all the necessary details, in respect of the deceased's date of birth, next-of-kin, religion and other demographic details are correct. They should also identify if the deceased had any implants of any kind so that the undertakers are made aware of them. The doctor, who has the responsibility for the signing of the death certificate, will need to know if the deceased is to be buried or cremated as there are different forms that need completing (www.direct.gov.uk 2009). An additional, independent doctor is required to sign cremation forms (Ministry of Justice, 2008) and this can cause delays in issuing the paperwork to relatives. Waiting for a confirmatory death certificate, which starts the process of registering the death, the issuing of a final death certificate and the funeral arrangements, can often be a fraught experience for the relatives. The UK Government issues a free booklet entitled 'What to do after a death' (www.direct.gov.uk 2009) that specifies that registering a death needs to take place within five days if it occurs in England, Wales or Northern Ireland or within eight days in Scotland. Other countries, outside the UK, will have similar guidelines or policies.

Those patients who have made a will may have considered whether they want a burial or a cremation (or even to donate their body to medical science).

Table 16.1 Major religions and aspects of the dying phase and funerals

Religion	Timing of ceremony	Burial or cremation	Days of mourning	Other information
Christian	No set time	Burial or cremation	None set	• Dark clothes normally worn • May be a wake as part of the ceremony • May be a memorial service later
Jewish	Within 24 hours	Burial	Year of official mourning	• Have a burial society *Chevra Kadisha*, who prepare the body for burial • Symbolic tear in clothes (indicating broken heart) • In the first week there is a *shiva,* where the family initially mourn alone. After 4 days friends and acquaintances visit the mourners at home
Hindu	No set time	Cremation	13 days	• May want to die on the floor, in contact with the earth • Relatives may not want to touch the dying person • Eldest male chief mourner – may shave their head as a mark of respect • White is worn
Sikh	No set time	Cremation	Between 2 and 5 weeks	• Mourners are quiet – emotions kept controlled • Ashes scattered in sea or running water
Islam	Within 24 hours	Buried, on their right side, facing *Makkah* (Mecca) Cremation is forbidden	3 days, or longer for remaining spouse	• Body wrapped in simple white shroud • Ritual washing of the body by family members, who are the same sex as the deceased • May not use a coffin
Buddhist	No set time	Cremation favoured	None set but there is a belief that the spirit is reborn after 49 days	• No set traditions, as the physical body is considered a shell, but a photograph of the person may be displayed • White clothing and headbands may be worn

Source: www.ifishoulddie.co.uk (2009b)

For others their religious beliefs may dictate what follows (see Table 16.1). These long-established rituals remain the main template for today's funerals. However, if the patient does not follow a religious practice, then there are alternative funeral services, for example, of a Humanist funeral or a civil funeral. The excellent website www.ifishoulddie.co.uk (2009a) states that 'Humanist non-religious funeral ceremonies acknowledge loss and celebrate a life without employing religious rituals' while a Civil funeral is defined as: 'A funeral, which is driven by the wishes, beliefs and values of the deceased and their family, not by the beliefs or ideology of the person conducting the funeral.' Funeral directors generally have information about persons within the locality who are able to lead such services. In addition, funeral directors are able to give information and advice on alternative types of burial such as woodland burials, and different types of coffins such as those made of wicker or eco-pods.

The decision about which type of funeral to have may well rest on the financial status of the deceased and their family. There may be disagreements within the family about how much to spend, with 'plain and simple' – for example, basic coffin, no flowers and no extra cars – being at one end of the continuum to 'spare no expense' – with finest coffin, high cost venue, and musicians – at the other end. This aspect is especially an issue for families where there is a reliance on the state benefit system, such as those with young families (Cordon et al., 2001).

The patient, prior to death, may be aware of these issues and may wish to discuss them with healthcare staff. The palliative care stage of life may be the time that patients actively engage with the planning of their funerals. Articulating and identifying advance funeral wishes can alleviate much of the anxiety and there exists plans, as exemplified in *The Natural Death Handbook* (Wienrich and Speyer, 2003), that enable this process. Charities such as Age Concern and Cruse Bereavement Care also promote the notion of advanced planning for funerals to cut down on unnecessary costs and family discord. The 'What to do after a death' booklet also gives information about death grants and benefits.

A potential area for family discord and discussion is the presence of children at a funeral. In Victorian times children would probably have witnessed a death in the immediate family. Illustrations of funerals of that period, though, often show children as bystanders rather than part of the funeral procession (May, 2003). During the early twentieth century children were mostly excluded from funeral services but towards the end of the century grief in children was acknowledged (Worden, 1996) and now more thought is given to having children attend and participate in the service. This is especially important where the deceased is a child, for example, a sibling or school-friend. With education about the funeral process, through talking and perhaps using photographs, and support from family and friends, attendance need not be any more stressful than it is for adult attendees. In fact, children may actually bring light relief to an otherwise very emotional day. They can be encouraged to write a memorial poem or start a memory box (Wienrich and Speyer, 2003) in order to have an outlet for their grief. Many hospices provide bereavement care and counsellors often have the skills to aid discussions with parents of young and teenage children.

Healthcare professionals in other settings may find it useful to find out what is available in their area in order to support the patients and families at this difficult time.

PRACTICAL APPLICATION OF THE CONCEPT

Margaret was dying from ovarian cancer. She had received several cycles of chemotherapy so she knew that time was limited. She discussed her funeral with her husband and as she had no particular faith, she stated she did not want a religious service. She asked to be cremated so that she would be near to where her parents' ashes were scattered, in the grounds of a local crematorium. After her death her husband tried to comply with his wife's wishes and asked family members to officiate.

However, they declined, acknowledging that they would be too upset to shoulder the responsibility. Consequently he contacted a vicar to lead the service, who delivered a very traditional belief-based eulogy, contrary to Margaret's final wishes. Had Margaret or her husband had more information about the types of funeral that are available, it might have prevented the anguish experienced by her husband and other relatives. However, her granddaughter, aged 8, attended the funeral and placed a flower on the coffin at the end of the service.

See also: *loss, grief and bereavement*

FURTHER READING

Walters, T. (1994) *The Revival of Death*. London: Routledge.
Wienrich, S. and Speyer, J. (2003) *Natural Death Handbook*, 4th edn. London: Random House.
Which? Essential Guides (2009) *What to Do When Someone Dies: From Funeral Planning to Probate and Finance*. Worthing: Which? Books.

REFERENCES

Corden, A., Sloper, P. and Sainsbury, R. (2001) 'Financial effects for families after the death of a disabled or chronically ill child: a neglected dimension of bereavement', *Child Care, Health & Development*, 28(3): 199–204.
May, T. (2003) *The Victorian Undertaker*. Risborough: Shire Publications Ltd.
Ministry of Justice (2008) *Cremation Regulations 2008: Guidance for Doctors*. Available at: www.justice.gov.uk, accessed 6 August 2009.
Wienrich, S. and Speyer, J. (2003) *Natural Death Handbook*, 4th edn. London: Random House.
Worden, J.W. (1996) *Children and Grief: When a Parent Dies*. New York: Guilford Press
www.askoxford.com (2009) 'Funeral', accessed 5 August 2009.
www.direct.gov.uk (2009) 'What to do after a death', accessed 6 August 2009.
www.ifishoulddie.co.uk (2009a) 'Non-religious alternatives', accessed 5 August 2009.
www.ifishoulddie.co.uk (2009b) 'Religious traditions and beliefs', accessed 5 August 2009.

17 good death

Moyra A. Baldwin and Jan Woodhouse

DEFINITION

If each of us was to ask all those we know what they believe a good death is, there would be as many variations as the people giving their opinions, dependent on the person's age, history, presence or absence of illness, culture, experience, and a whole range of other factors. There is no clear definition of the concept good death but that is not necessarily unique, as there are several similarly difficult to define concepts in palliative care, as many chapters in this book discuss. Good death has been studied and discussed from patients' and healthcare professionals' perspectives, from hospice and community settings, as well as across cultures and communities. While 'a good death has no universal definition' (Hattori et al., 2006: 169), what is slightly clearer is the notion that one's perception of a good death is unique to each one, and may well be a dynamic concept for the patient, family and healthcare professional, alike.

KEY POINTS

- A good death is a concept that each of us defines differently.
- There are both common and contentious components of a good death.
- Pain and symptom management are essential components of a good death.

DISCUSSION

Hattori et al. (2006: 169) concluded their concept analysis study of good death in a Japanese community claiming that a 'universal definition' was not available. Using a well-recognised method of concept analysis the authors identified a list of 20 surrogate terms that were drawn from the disciplines of nursing, medicine, anthropology and sociology. Among the 20, examples of terms associated with good death included a correct death, happy, gradual and sudden death. From these four alternatives it can be seen that good death has a range of meanings, some even appearing the opposite of others. Based on the attributes of a good death, the authors, nevertheless, proposed that a good death was 'a multi-dimensional, ceaseless individual experience based on personal and socio-cultural domains of life that incorporate the person's past

good death

77

present and future' (Hattori et al., 2006: 167). It is with the individual aspect of the concept that this chapter will explore good death.

Weisman's notion of an 'appropriate death' takes account of the individual. Weisman (1988) introduced the term 'appropriate death' as one of three key areas that a hospice programme should include and noted that 'obviously an appropriate death for one person may be unsuitable for another. What might seem appropriate from the outside might be utterly meaningless to the dying person himself. Conversely, deaths that seem unacceptable to an outsider might be desirable from the inner viewpoint of the patient.' Thus it is evident, that for a good death, palliative care professionals needs to consider the individual patient facing death and avoid making assumptions about what constitutes a good death.

Good death

Having been explored from a range of stances including professionals, dying people and their families and in various settings, the bereaved family, as well as from the context of different cultures, one might expect that good death is a well-defined concept. There are common features in some explorations, for example, pain control, dignity, choice of location of dying and support for spiritual, psychosocial and emotional needs (see Table 17.1). Others, however, are notably different and some, even, potentially contentious. Being able to exercise control over one's dying and death has, as Age Concern (2008) notes, introduced ethical dimensions to good death which render it a contentious issue for contemporary palliative care.

Steinhauser et al. (2000) explored the concept in their study using a grounded theory approach, which elicited six components of a good death. The 75 participants comprised patients, family members, and healthcare providers from hospitals and hospices in USA (Steinhauser et al., 2000). The researchers explored the experiences of deaths of family members, friends and patients using focus groups over a period of four months to identify what made the deaths good or bad. The findings included pain and symptom management, clear decision-making, preparation for death, completion, contributing to others and affirmation of whole person.

Clearly, pain and symptom management are key and common components of a good death (Table 17.1): Age Concern (1999, 2008), Mak and Clinton (1999), Vig et al., (2002), and Miyashita et al. (2008) identify these aspects. Not all studies, however, note clear decision-making as explicitly as Steinhauser et al. (2000) yet there is an implication that decision-making is essential to patient empowerment. Patients' fear of pain and poor symptom management, along with families' needs to have their concerns listened to, require clarity in respect of decision-making in order that pain and other distressing symptoms can be managed effectively and crises avoided.

An important component of a good death, for some, is preparation for the approaching death (Age Concern 1999; Mak and Clinton, 1999). The individual

Table 17.1 Concept of a good death

Age Concern (1999 and 2008)	Mak and Clinton (1999)	Steinhauser et al. (2000)	Vig et al. (2002)	Hattori et al. (2006)	Miyashita et al. (2008)
Know when death is coming and understand what can be expected	Comfort or relief from pain and suffering	Pain and symptom management	Avoidance of pain	Socio-cultural norms including past, present and future	Comfort – environmental, physical and psychological
Retain control of what happens	Openness or being aware of dying	Clear decision-making	Quickly without suffering	Personal experience	Life completion
Dignity and privacy	Completion or accepting the timing of one's death	Preparation for death	Without knowledge of impending death	Multi-dimensional and continuous process	Dying in a favourite place
Have control over pain relief and other symptom control	Control or acceptance and autonomy	Completion			Maintaining hope and pleasure
Have choice and control over where death occurs	Optimism or keeping hope alive	Contributing to others			Good relationships with medical staff and family
Access to information and expertise	Readiness or preparing for departure	Affirmation of whole person			Not being a burden to others
Access to spiritual or emotional support	Location, living with choice about where to die				Respected as an individual
Access to hospice care in any location					
Control over who is present and who shares the end					
Issue advance directives which ensure wishes are respected					

(Continued)

Table 17.1   (Continued)

Age Concern (1999 and 2008)	Mak and Clinton (1999)	Steinhauser et al. (2000)	Vig et al. (2002)	Hattori et al. (2006)	Miyashita et al. (2008)
Time to say goodbye, and control over other aspects of timing					
Leave when it is time to go, and not have life prolonged pointlessly					

nature of this perception was clearly to be seen in Britain in the last century, for example, people who lived in cramped accommodation might be concerned about the width of the stairs if they were narrow, as bringing the coffin down, following a death in the family, would be a challenge. There is also a long history of preparing for death by the purchase of a plot in a cemetery along with preparations for the funeral. Vig et al. (2002) found that a good death for 4 of the 16 patients in their study was one that did not include knowledge of the impending death. These patients, while not dying, were considered to be at increased risk of death because of their history of cancer, heart problems, or both, which may explain the findings. One patient, however, identified a bad death as one in which there was knowledge of the death. Clearly, for some it is important to be prepared for death, for others, preparation for death is less desirable.

The seminal works on 'awareness' contexts (Glaser and Strauss, 1965) and the 'acceptance' stage of dying (Kübler-Ross, 1969) reflect the essence of preparing for the final event. Similarly, the patients and families in the study by Steinhauser et al. (2000) wanted to know what to expect during the illness trajectory and prepare for events after the death, such as planning the funeral. These aspects also relate to the 'completion' in the study by Steinhauser et al. (2000). Enabling patients and their families to address unfinished business prior to death is, indeed, a common component of health and social care professionals' work in palliative care and might encompass, for example, psycho-social, spiritual, or legal aspects which individuals want to complete before their death.

'Contributing to others' and 'affirmation of the whole person', the two remaining components in the Steinhauser et al. (2000) study, they claim, have not previously been identified. While this may be so there is ample evidence, every day, of patients contributing to others, for example, entering a clinical trial which may not offer any benefit to the patient but can offer hope for the future of others. Others contribute by running marathons or similarly long and enduring activities to raise money for the charity that closely relates to their illness. It may be that in doing so their contribution also enables them to be recognised as a 'unique and whole person'. This was important to the relatives in the Steinhauser et al. (2000) study and relates to the holistic and individualised concepts of care that are associated with palliative caring.

PRACTICAL APPLICATION OF THE CONCEPT

William and Betty, both in their late eighties, had suffered with heart failure and chronic obstructive pulmonary disease for years. They each spent frequent short-stay spells in hospital over the past two years and knew they were 'failing', as they told their family. Having enjoyed a happy life together, and being philosophical about death – most of their friends had died before them, they had planned for their dying, death and funeral, and wanted the family to know their wishes. Their two daughters, in their fifties, and the six grand-children aged between 16 and 30 were less happy to discuss their demise, but appreciated that for their mum and dad/grandpa a 'good death' meant that they had their wishes fulfilled. Between the hospital stays, physically, William's and Betty's medicines controlled symptoms. Psycho-socially they had prepared for their death by leaving important papers safely with each daughter. Their wills left legacies for the grand-children and each had written an advance directive. What they wanted most was to die at home because they knew the community nurses, the community team knew them and treated them as individuals with kindness and caring. A good death for William and Betty involved being prepared. Having their symptoms managed was important, as were making important decisions in preparation for death and afterwards, and contributing to their grand-children's future. Knowing that they could rely on their daughters and the healthcare professionals when the time came affirmed them as individuals and made them feel valued.

See also: attributes of palliative caring; holism

FURTHER READING

http://www.ifishoulddie.co.uk/

REFERENCES

Age Concern (1999) *Debate of the Age Health and Care Study Group. The Future of Health and Care of Older People: The Best is Yet to Come.* London: Age Concern.

Age Concern (2008) *Policy position papers: Dying and Death.* London: Age Concern. Available at: http://www.ageconcern.org.uk/AgeConcern/Documents/DyingandDeathppp Feb2008.pdf, accessed 21 September 2009.

Glaser, B.G. and Strauss, A.L. (1965) *Awareness of Dying.* Chicago: Aldine.

Hattori, K., McCubbin, M.A. and Ishida, D.N. (2006) 'Concept analysis of good death in the Japanese community', *Journal of Nursing Scholarship*, 38(20): 165–70.

Kübler-Ross, E. (1969) *On Death and Dying.* New York: Macmillan.

Mak, J.M.H. & Clinton, M. (1999) 'Promoting a good death: an agenda for outcomes research – a review of the literature', *Nursing Ethics*, 6(2): 97–106.

good death

Miyashita, M., Morita, T., Sato, K., Hirai, K., Shima, Y. and Uchitomi, Y. (2008) 'Factors contributing to evaluation of a good death from the bereaved family member's perspective', *Psycho-oncology*, 17: 612–20.

Steinhauser, K.E., Clipp, E.C., McNeilly, M., Christakis, N.A., McIntyre, L.M. and Tulsky, J.A. (2000) 'In search of a good death: observations of patients, families and providers', *Annals of Internal Medicine*, 132(10): 825–32.

Vig, E.K., Davenport, N.A. and Pearlman, R.A. (2002) 'Good deaths, bad deaths, and preferences for the end-of-life: a qualitative study of geriatric outpatients', *Journal of American Geriatrics Society*, 50(9): 1541–8.

Weisman, A.D. (1988) 'Appropriate death and the hospice program', *The Hospice Journal*, 4(1): 65–77.

18 the globalisation of palliative care

Lynda Prescott

DEFINITION

This chapter starts essentially by asking the question 'can or should we consider ourselves members of discrete society or are we all part of a world community?' Social life, the way in which humans are organised, roles, organisations, and institutions are the building blocks, and culture is the cement. Internationally the development of telecommunications and technology has led to a modification in culture and our expectations of how we communicate.

Globalisation, a broad societal force with deep implications, is a process through which people's lives become connected, economically, politically and culturally. Cultures have rarely been completely isolated from outside influences because throughout time people have been moving, trading goods and exchanging ideas. What is different in the twenty-first century is the speed and scope of communication and change.

'Spreading the word', about concepts relating to End of Life among a population who have become familiar with rapid change

Using information technology across the globe offers practitioners from all health professions a chance to learn from each other fast, for example, sharing advice when symptom management becomes complex. Additionally, access by the lay public, who often share the same information sites as the professional, provides powerful problem-solving solutions, and shared communication platforms provide opportunities to keep a finger on the societal pulse. Within the context of a receding global economy the need to communicate the concept of palliative care and the suggestion that palliative care services improve care and can save money has never been more pressing. Technology enables the global sharing of palliative care philosophy, and sound practice around end of life, including research within multi-professional groups.

As financial cutbacks affect the public health systems across the world and constrain traditional formal education and conference opportunities for health-care professionals (Ling, 2008), the dissemination of the identity, purpose, qualities and values associated with palliation requires creative thought. The need for flexibility of access, unification of voices and coordinated effort can, in part, be addressed by the adoption of electronic communication strategies.

Social constructivist theory suggests that relationships between individuals and society are reciprocal as we can modify roles, change norms and revolutionise institutions. The potential of a global, virtual, instant audience and a platform where death and dying can be discussed, may create a groundswell for reclamation of death as a natural process and the acceptance of palliative care philosophy within Western nations. A global communication method enables the sharing of alternative traditions around end of life.

KEY POINTS

- Twenty-first-century society is considered in global terms.
- The use of available technology enhances the opportunities available for sharing.
- Technology enables the sharing of associated cultural beliefs around death and dying.
- Within a context of global recession the need to espouse collaborative, flexible communication about palliative care is an imperative.
- In a competitive market there is a need for health professionals to ensure end of life care is not forgotten when decisions are made about expenditure.
- Information technology enables shared communication and across all stakeholders including powerful insights into patient and carer experiences.
- By generating discussion there is more opportunity for role and norms to be modified.

DISCUSSION

Palliative care is a poorly understood 'business' but technological advances have provided a catalyst for change by providing opportunities for review and reflection. Adopting electronic tools for communication provides a platform for understanding social psychology around death and dying from the perspective of patient, carer and health care professional. Viewing materials is straightforward and swift, often compelling and persuasive.

Google searching or using an academic search engine is often the first step in a process that reveals global information and discussion: websites and web casts bringing information together, enabling the exchange of conceptual models. Message boards and blogs offer tools and resources for collaboration. The major aims of such tools are the enablement of informed and competent decisions by all stakeholders in end-of-life care. Upon this platform shared meanings are explored and essential palliative care concepts agreed, for example goals of care, pain management strategies, medication protocols and care pathways. An example of this is the palliativedrugs.com website. The content is based on the UK Palliative Care Formulary (PCF3) (Twycross and Wilcock, 2007), the associated bulletin board enables health professionals to discuss drug and non-pharmaceutical issues and to problem solve. Postings and replies are from across professional groups and from all parts of the world.

For the lay carers the powerful expression of experiences in bite-size chunks provide insight into human experiences. Carers are active in the conveyance of their messages, frequently highlighting the disparities in care. Carers challenge the taboo surrounding death, highlighting the right to choose treatment options including the place of death. The medicalisation of death is challenged, for example, zangani.com offers support to the hospice service promotion of The Palliative Care (Scotland) Bill (2008) providing a forum for carers to advocate for better end of life care while highlighting emerging palliative care needs for those with chronic diseases, such as heart failure, renal failure and dementia. Each segment of video highlights the need for living and dying well, creating an opportunity to share carer perspectives with health professionals and policy-makers.

For health professionals the Internet offers opportunities to share, using a wide variety of communication strategies from online academic publications, web-based surveys and bulletin boards for information exchange, web and podcasts. An example is http://www.palliative.info, based in Canada (Harlos, 2009). Led by a medical professor the site offers teaching materials and local and global information. The nursing profession appears to have adopted pod and video web-cast to explore palliative care in the context of twenty first century nursing an example would be http://www.nursetv.com (Nurse TV Community Television Project, 2009). The website format offers a story-telling approach as a way to share information and experiences plus a blog for further discussion.

Hall (2009) considers nursing students as a group who access technology for both information and entertainment. The emerging generation of nurses is perceived as being open to collaboration: comfortable with online tools they come to expect openness and innovation. Within the context of palliative care, nursing forums are discussing nursing competency, and levels of skill and knowledge are explored in the light of emerging nursing philosophy. Nurse

TV (Australia) is a site where palliative care is discussed using a combination of community television and YouTube. This strategy utilises a carer perspective as a mechanism to review care received from palliative care teams and to outline the role of the nurse.

For policy-makers, technology provides an insight into cultural change and public perceptions. For health academics, there are opportunities to explore topics that are open for discussion and to share research findings. For researchers and policy-makers, there are forums where they are able to consider concerns about providing palliative care for an aging population. The cost and availability of services for those with chronic disease as well as cancer are projected and open for discussion among all stakeholders. Electronic tools enable the sharing of these projections and concerns, enabling discussion and potential problem-solving. An example of this would be the Palliative Care Policy Centre (http://www.medicaring.org/) from the United States. Lynn and Adamson (2003) suggest that 'the baby boomers' will find it difficult to find care as so many will live with chronic disease towards the end of their lives. This situation may create a burden for potential family carers, who are projected to be fewer in number due to demographic change.

The ideal of compassionate, competent end-of-life care is expounded across the lifespan. Various patterns of death, and related difficulties in predicting death trajectories, highlight the need for further global exploration and research. Within the context of minority groups, those imprisoned and in marginalised groups, such as those in Angola, Louisiana's infamous maximum-security prison, are among the unlikeliest to achieve an end-of-life success. The institution is home for over five thousand inmates who are expected to grow old and die behind bars, with few gaining parole before death. The adoption of palliative care principles, symptom management including counselling, provides a microcosm open to research, into the value of adopting a palliative care philosophy. In turn, the emerging philosophy is shared, using the internet, with published papers available online.

In the technological media there is an attempt to understand a social tension between care givers, who have concerns about dashing hope and the creation of despair. Alongside chat room evidence, it suggests that the first question asked, of those diagnosed with terminal illness, is about death. Feedback via blogs and bulletin boards suggest that this is a global phenomenon. Furthermore, the challenges surrounding death and the perception of palliative care, need to be considered in terms of a social construct over time, experiences and mores.

Technological advances have enabled a significant proportion of the world to communicate more efficiently, but to view information technology as a panacea resolving problems with end of life care would be a mistake. No other medium can match television for the size of its audience. For example, as of September 1, 2008, there was an estimated 114.5 million households in the United States (Wikipedia, 2008). Within the UK context television is the main source of accessing national and world news and entertainment for nearly 70% of consumers. TV is also the medium that 55 per cent of people would miss most if it were removed (Ofcom, 2008). The medium of television has been used to create social interaction, in the form of discussion. Adopting 'soap opera' storylines, difficult and sometimes challenging aspects of palliative care, including barriers and the political firestorm of euthanasia and physician assisted suicide have been played out. Thus watching TV is an enabler for socializing. Gossiping about plotlines and being up-to-date with a programme is a form of social currency, and it therefore provides an arena for discussing death and potentially removes the taboo.

There is an emerging convergence of media as consumers of all ages display a growing interest in accessing audio-visual content online (Ofcom, 2008). There are clear opportunities to harness documented consumer enthusiasm for the new converging media to promote communication and mutual support within the context of the intimate human experience of dying. However a lot of people feel overwhelmed by the amount of choice available. One of the major criticisms of complex contemporary communication media is its dehumanising form. The maximization of efficiency has a cost. Hall (2009) suggests that rather than using multimedia, as a replacement for face-to-face interaction, there is a desire for a blend of communication strategies. This is an important consideration, as social structures such as palliative care require constant human support. Once we, as a society, are no longer able to sustain organisations, such as the hospice, or believe in our institutions, they fall apart.

PRACTICAL APPLICATION OF THE CONCEPT

The Canadian Virtual Hospice (Chochinov and Cory, 2009) is an easily accessible globally available resource. Within the site there is a variety of resources for both the lay public and health professionals. The use of storytelling from carers enables the sharing of personal experience with a global audience. The families take their place as the experts on living through death, providing professionals and policy-makers with an insight into the social construction of death and dying and what contributes to a good death.

The digital age allows one to reach inside human experiences that are intimate by offering opportunities for communication and mutual support. The insights provided can be shared with individuals, multi-professional associations, policy-makers and business.

See also: communication; information technology

FURTHER READING

Asthana, A. and Thorpe, V. (2005) 'Whatever happened to the original Generation X?'. *The Observer*, 23 January. Available at: http://www.guardian.co.uk/uk/2005/jan/23/british identity.anushkaasthana, accessed 14 September 2009.
Palliative Care Policy Centre (2009) *About PCPC*, available at: www.medicaring.org/, accessed 14 September 2009.

REFERENCES

Chochinov, H.M. and Cory, S. (Executives) (2009) *Canadian Virtual Hospital*, available at: www.virtualhospice.ca, accessed 14 September 2009.

Hall, HW.A. (2009) 'Whither nursing education? Possibilities, panaceas and problems', *Nurse Education Today*, 29(3): 268–75.

Harlos, M. (2009) Palliative care links and resource material, available at: www.palliative. info, accessed 14 September 2009.

Ling, J. (2008) 'Palliative care in changing economic times', *International Journal of Palliative Nursing*, 14(11): 523–25.

Lynn, A. and Adamson, D. M. (2003) *Living Well at the End of Life: Adapting Health Care to Serious Chronic Illness in Old Age*. Santa Monica: Rand.

Nurse TV Community Television Project (2009) *Nurse TV (Australia)*, available at: www. nursesandmidwives.com/nurse-tv, accessed 14 September 2009.

Ofcom (2008) The Communications Market 2008, available at: www.ofcom.org.uk/ research/cm/cmr08/, accessed 14 September 2009.

Twycross, R. and Wilcock, A. (eds) (2007) Palliative drugs.com Ltd, available at: www.palliativedrugs.com/, accessed 14 September 2009.

Palliative Care(Scotland) Bill (2008), available at: www.zangani.com, accessed 14 September 2009.

19 holism

Moyra A. Baldwin and Joanne Greenwood

DEFINITION

The concept holism has a long history. The noun 'holism' and adjective 'holistic' are reported to have been first used by the South African philosopher Smuts in 1926 (Ham-Ying, 1993). Ham-Ying's (1993) analysis of the concept holism notes that it is derived from the Greek 'holos' which means 'whole'. Holism in the context of health and social care means caring for the 'whole' person. The entire person is more than a collection of unrelated systems or symptoms. Holistic care involves practitioners responding in a way that acknowledges that the 'whole is greater than the sum of its parts'. A definition of holism therefore concerns the multi-dimensional aspect of people. Individuals are not simply made of separate physical, psychological, spiritual, social, cultural or emotional dimensions but all of these, working and interacting as an integrated whole. Working to this philosophy, holism and holistic care have become associated with hospice and palliative care.

KEY POINTS

- Holism relates to the whole person.
- Holism and reductionism are not mutually exclusive but require integration.
- Holism incorporates elements that relate to both patients and practitioners.

DISCUSSION

Holism relates to the whole person

The National Institute for Health and Clinical Excellence [NICE] (2004: 20) acknowledges that the principles of palliative care incorporate holism, defining palliative care as 'active holistic care' and guiding healthcare professionals to understand that palliative care aims to 'integrate the psychological and spiritual aspects of patient care'. Palliative care includes promoting the physical and emotional well-being of patients facing life-limiting illness and fundamental, to the process, is the relationship between palliative care practitioner and the patient.

Holism is a philosophical view of the person that encompasses physical, psychological, spiritual, social, cultural and emotional aspects. According to Buckley (2002), however, this common definition overlooks an essential component of holism. At the 'heart of holism', Buckley (2002) notes, is the use of the person's own innate resources and this applies to both the patient and practitioner. As noted above and in other chapters, the philosophy of palliative care and holism are closely linked. To provide excellence in palliative care the professional carer needs to be able to engage with patients and their families in such a way as to build a confident and trusting relationship. This demonstrates a caring approach to the person's suffering. It is an holistic, 'whole', or total care approach to people whose needs are regarded as more than the sum of the suffering associated with the individual symptoms, distress or a specific illness label.

Holism and reductionism are not mutually exclusive but require integration

Griffin (1993) reminds one that holism has a positive inference. It is the opposite of fragmentation and impersonalisation which was seen in an over-specialised healthcare world at the time. The same may be said today as reductionistic approaches to healthcare can detract from holistic health and well-being. Advances in technology and increasing emphasis on evidence-based treatments and management could result in approaching a person's healthcare problem from a single, reductionistic, perspective and may be detrimental the person's whole well-being. Nevertheless, Pietroni (1997) offers a note of caution regarding the negative inference associated with reductionism, on the one hand, and the positive presumption with holism on the other. To be able to practise holistically, he argues, one needs to consider the reductionist perspective. One such reductionistic, or singular, aspect of palliative care we can consider is physical symptoms, and how they relate to the whole. For example, when a person feels physical pain, there are likely to be other, similarly singular, elements associated with the pain experience, such as psychological, emotional, social, spiritual or cultural pain issues. Take the case of a patient who has a cancer diagnosis and who is experiencing physical pain. The physical pain felt may be magnified by the meaning the person attaches to it and, in this case, it may be that the person's pain includes worrying about whether the cancer has spread. The pain experience for this person will include not only the singular physical but other similarly singular elements, namely, psychological and emotional. In Pietroni's (1997) terms *all* the singular, or reductionistic, elements need consideration if the person's pain is to be managed effectively. Thus holism enhances reductionism by giving consideration to the relationship between the parts, in this way the person is viewed and cared for as an integrated whole whose symptoms and needs are interdependent, not disconnected elements. Table 19.1 presents the principles of holism and holistic care.

Holism incorporates elements that relate to both patients and practitioners

Founded in 1983, the British Holistic Medical Association (BHMA) (Holmes 1984) noted that holism comprised four principles:

1 Responding to the person as a whole in his/her environment.
2 Willingness to use a wide range of orthodox and complementary interventions.
3 Encouraging individual self-responsibility.
4 Recognising the importance of the practitioner's own health.

Table 19.1 Holism, principles of holism and holistic care

Ham-Ying (1993) Holism	BHMA (2009) Principles of holism	Griffin (1993) Holistic care
Person as a total/whole being	Responding to the person as a whole in his/her environment	Respect for persons
Identification of dimensions and systems which make up the whole	Willingness to use a wide a range of orthodox and complementary interventions	Openness and receptivity
Relationship between parts and between parts and the whole	Encouraging individual self-responsibility	Reflection
Whole is greater than the sum of its parts	Recognising the importance of the practitioner's own health	Seeing comprehensively

The BHMA's core values which the association claims underpin holistic practice include compassion, respect, open-mindedness, competence, and self-care (bhma.org, 2009). It is evident, then, that holism is not simply about the care of patients and their families: it also concerns the practitioner: a point noted in the study conducted by Davies and Oberle (1990). 'Preserving own integrity' recognises the importance of the professional carer's own health.

Ham-Ying (1993) noted this in her concept analysis in which she clarified holism as a view of the person, which equates with the discussion above, and as an approach to the delivery of nursing care. As an approach to care delivery, the antecedents noted by Ham-Ying (1993) included the carer having possession of knowledge, skills, attitudes and other resources to enable delivery of appropriate care. These are similar to the preconditions of holistic caring that Griffin (1993) identified in her exploration of holism in nursing. Practitioners who claim that they provide holistic care demonstrate attitudes and values that incorporate respect, receptivity, reflection, and the ability to see comprehensively. These, according to Griffin (1993), are a necessity if we are to understand the uniqueness of humans. Holism, holistic caring and holistic palliative care are depicted diagrammatically, and holistically, in Figure 19.1 (Holism and Palliative Care). Holism in the context of palliative care addresses the unique, and individual, nature of the person acknowledging integration and interdependence of the physical, psychological, spiritual, social, cultural and emotional parts. Consideration of these singular elements is important to achieve holistic palliative care. The holistic practitioner respects the individuality of the person, is receptive to the person's palliative care needs, reflects on these to provide effective care and management, and comprehensively considers a wide range of options. Applying these aspects of holism to palliative care requires recognition of the integration of living with and dying from a life-limiting illness.

PRACTICAL APPLICATION OF THE CONCEPT

Jean, admitted to the hospice for complex symptom management, was in the terminal phase of her illness. Following Jean's divorce from her husband who was the father of her daughter Hannah, Jean developed a long-term partnership with Joanna, and they lived together for eight years. Joanna was her named next of kin and was a constant visitor to the hospice, sharing Jean's room almost all day and all night. Hannah found her mother's relationship with Joanna distressing and she resented her presence at her mother's bedside.

Working to the philosophy of palliative the hospice staff were pleased with the success of Jean's physical symptom management. Practising holistic palliative care they supported Jean and Joanna, and Hannah recognising that each had physical, psychological, emotional, social, spiritual and cultural needs that influenced both the suffering and comfort they were experiencing. They respected Jean's relationship with her partner, as well as Hannah's feeling of hurt and betrayal, and Joanna's need to be with her partner during the

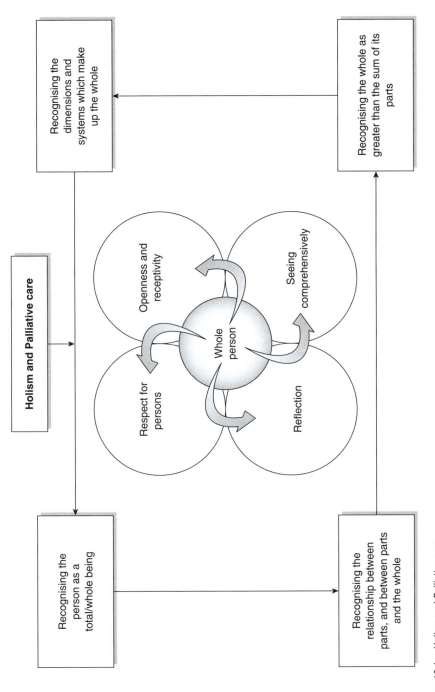

Figure 19.1 *Holism and Palliative care*
Source: BHMA (2009), Griffin (1993), and Ham-Ying (1993)

dying phase of Jean's life. They empathised with Joanna and Hannah, receptive to their needs considering the options available to support them while Jean was terminally ill. They provided holistic support to both Joanna and Hannah preparing them for the time when Jean died and ensured they would receive bereavement support appropriate to their needs.

See also: attributes of palliative caring

FURTHER READING

www.bhma.org

REFERENCES

BHMA (2009) BHMA core values, available at: www.bhma.org/new_site/values.php, accessed 5 October 2009.

Buckley, J. (2002) 'Holism and a health-promoting approach to palliative care', *International Journal of Palliative Nursing*, 8(10): 505–8.

Davies, B., and Oberle, K. (1990) 'Dimensions of the supportive role of the nurse in palliative care', *Oncology Nursing Forum*, 17(1): 87–94.

Griffin, A. (1993) 'Holism in nursing: its meaning and value', *British Journal of Nursing*, 2(6): 310–12.

Ham-Ying, S. (1993) 'Analysis of the concept holism within the context of nursing', *British Journal of Nursing*, 2(15): 771–5.

Holmes, P. (1984) 'Holistic nursing', *Nursing Times*, 80: 28–9.

National Institute for Health and Clinical Excellence (NICE) (2004) *Improving Supportive and Palliative Care for Adults with Cancer*. London: NICE.

Pietroni, P. (1997) 'Is complementary medicine holistic?', *Complementary Therapies in Nursing & Midwifery*, 3: 9–11.

key concepts in palliative care

92

20 hospice movement and evolution of palliative care

Moyra A. Baldwin

DEFINITION

The modern hospice movement in its early form in the 1960s, its development to palliative and specialist palliative care during the 1980s, and to end of life care in the first decade of the twenty-first century demonstrates the evolution of palliative care over a period of half a century. Palliative care from its inception and delivery in hospices continues to provide and promote quality of life and living for people who have life-limiting illnesses. The early modern hospices provided care for people, usually adults, diagnosed with a cancer whereas contemporary palliative care includes care of people of all ages, and their families, where the patient has a diagnosis of a life-limiting illness other than cancer. Palliative care has evolved to enable quality of life, quality of living and quality of dying across a range of health, social and home care settings, provided by a multi-disciplinary team including professionals, volunteers and lay carers.

KEY POINTS

- Hospice and Palliative care espouse quality of life for the dying person, individuality for the patient and family, and potential for growth in suffering.
- Palliative care has evolved from a service based in hospices to a multi-disciplinary community-wide service incorporating both orthodox and complementary interventions.
- Palliative care has reached a degree of maturity, witnessed by critiques and challenges raised by a consumer-led society.

DISCUSSION

The concept of modern hospice which can be simply described as principles or a philosophy of care for the dying person, since its inception, has gathered momentum to such an extent that today it is a movement incorporating palliative care across the world. There is a much longer history to the modern hospice movement than the opening of St Christopher's in Sydenham in 1967. For Clark (2008), this was the culmination of the first phase of advancement of international palliative care. This chapter will explore the hospice movement and evolution of palliative care as a continuum of development and maturity: from the relative uncritical acceptance of the recent or modern hospice movement as an exemplary method of caring for the dying person and the patient's family to a greater willingness to offer critical comment on and to challenge contemporary palliative care philosophy.

Concept of modern hospice and palliative care – the WHO philosophy

The concept hospice resulted from the recognition of the neglect of terminally ill people being cared for in a health service that tended to abandon the dying. The early and enduring definition of hospice was captured by Saunders's (1978) philosophy of enabling people to live with a degree of quality to their life until they died and, when the time came, to die peacefully and in dignity. Hospices thus encompassed a positive attitude towards people who had a diagnosis of cancer so that they could live until death. Between Saunders's published philosophy and the World Health Organisation's (WHO) (1990) well-known definition (referred to in several chapters in this book) were other notable characterisations of hospice care, espousing individuality in living through a humanistic approach to care that addressed the bio-psycho-social needs of the person with a diagnosis of malignancy, and included care of the patient's family. Succinctly, Hanratty's (1989: 3) concept of hospice care demanded compassion, competence and constant attention to detail. By such means, and throughout the time of the patient's dying experience, the patient and family could have opportunities for growth and relief of suffering. Death is recognised as an inevitable part of life and there is willingness to discuss issues relating to dying and death. The nature of palliative care thus captures unique and individualised care of family units.

Changes in health and social care policy and, subsequently, the organisation of care delivery over the years have seen palliative care being introduced into a variety of care settings. Palliative care has spread from the hospice building into hospitals, community, nursing and residential homes, so that today it is delivered in urban, rural and remote settings. The palliative care team has similarly evolved to incorporate a range of health and social care professionals whose responsibility is to work and learn together to provide responsive comfort and care for its clients (Speck, 2006). Both traditional evidence-based and complementary therapeutic interventions aim to eradicate patients' pain and distressing symptoms. The palliative care team's focus is to provide holistic care and, to do this each discipline needs to know its role and the role of others in the team. This way, the team remains faithful to the philosophy of palliative care that was envisaged by the pioneers of the modern hospice movement.

Contrary to the presumption that a hospice is the place where people might want to die, it has been accepted by practitioners and Healthcare commissioners, operating in twenty-first century UK, that patients prefer to be cared for and to die at home. Government initiatives have subsequently focused on improving care for people facing the end of their lives (Department of Health, 2003; NICE, 2004) and achievement of a Gold Standard Framework (Thomas, 2003). Guidance has included improving supportive and palliative care and identifying people's preferences and priorities about the type and location of their end of life care. In 2008, the Department of Health anticipated that there would be greater choice in respect of where people wished to live and die, irrespective of their diagnosis (Department of Health, 2008). The strategy endorses a decrease in the number of emergency admissions to hospitals particularly when patients have expressly wished to die at home, and a reduction in the number of patients being transferred from a care home to a hospital in the last week of life. The emphasis is clearly on community palliative care.

The modern hospice movement and palliative care, initially considered to be care required when cure was no longer possible, has evolved into a continuum of care from the time of the patient's diagnosis and inevitable death to the family's care in their grief and bereavement. The addition of a diagnosis other than cancer, screening and investigations are extensions to the continuum which are supportive care throughout the illness trajectory, and life-maintaining care depicted in the Sheffield model (cited by Sutherland and Stevens, 2008). Palliative care is thus well established, moving away from terminal illness with a hospice connotation to be recognised as palliative care, a professional medical speciality in 1987 by the Royal College of Physicians, and advanced now by the UK government as an exemplar of end-of-life care. This might suggest that the evolution of the modern hospice movement and palliative care is without its critics but that is not the whole story.

Reconciling different perceptions

Randall and Downie (2006) identify a number of paradoxes in the palliative care philosophy, ranging from the discrepancy between developing evidence-based quantifiable tools to measure outcomes of qualitative concepts, to the specious emphasis on caring, equally, for the patient and family. Randall and Downie's (2006: 5) careful, constructive critique of the hospice evolution suggests that the transition to specialist palliative care has lost the original philosophy, having become 'too elaborate, too intrusive, too precious'. At the beginning of this chapter I noted that palliative care has evolved to enable 'quality of life, living and of dying'. Randall and Downie maintain that quality of life should not be a goal of palliative care not least because of its intricate and complex nature, and that it is almost impossible to define (see Randall and Downie, 2006, for a detailed discussion). If one accepts, however, that palliative care does improve quality of life the authors go on to question whether palliative care does this more so, and more cost-effectively, than traditional mainstream healthcare services. Nevertheless the modern hospice movement started because of uncaring and inhumane treatment of people at the end of life as noted above. It was, indeed, about quality of life which, at the time, mainstream healthcare failed to achieve.

Challenges

There are other challenges, too, that face the palliative care practitioner, some which appear to align with more of Randall and Downie's (2006) critique, for example, consumerism and responsibility. An example of the power of consumerism and rights-based individualism that has gathered momentum is the Royal College of Nursing's abandonment of its long-standing opposition to assisted suicide. This is in order that its members can openly debate euthanasia. Euthanasia, in other words, easeful death, could be considered as every palliative care practitioner's concern. Is it, though, a case that future evolvement of palliative care will be more than debating the issue of assisted suicide but practicing euthanasia? The concern for some practitioners, however, will be that the easeful death demanded by the consumer will mean more than palliation and symptom management. The worry will be that it will entail a deliberate act of symptom relief by killing the patient. I am only a little reassured by Randall and Downie's (2006) words that while the patient is the customer and consumer, the responsibility for the treatment or care *remains* with the professionals. The future may see continued demand to stray from the original hospice philosophy. The challenge for future healthcare commissioners procuring palliative care will be balancing patients', families' and lay and professional carers' competing demands.

PRACTICAL APPLICATION OF THE CONCEPT

As a student nurse in the 1970s working on my first placement, a surgical ward, I nursed Mr Markham who suffered a lot of pain. At the time and on reflection, the medical staff never believed that his pain was as bad as he said it was. Sadly, my memory of Mr Markham is of him asking for 'pain killers' but never having his suffering relieved by adequate analgesics. Post-mortem showed that he had cancer of the head of pancreas, known to be a painful condition. Had he been a patient today, his symptoms would have been investigated possibly as an out-patient, a team of palliative care professionals would have been involved advising on pain and symptom management commensurate with the severity of his suffering. His preferred priority/place of care and dying would have been ascertained, thus allowing him to be cared for at home, in hospital or in a hospice, and his wife may have been supported during his illness and after his death. What type of future service might be provided for Mr Markham or similar patients is hard to say but he could be one whose end-of-life care priority would be an easeful death – to die in dignity at a time and manner of his choosing.

See also: *legal and ethical issues; organisational management of palliative care; patient choice and preferences*

FURTHER READING

Clark, D. (2008) 'History and culture in the rise of palliative care', in S. Payne, J. Seymour and C. Ingleton (eds), *Palliative Care Nursing: Principles and Evidence for Practice*, 2nd edn. Maidenhead: McGraw-Hill/Open University Press, pp. 34–54.

Knight, A. (2001) 'Great Britain', in B.R. Ferrell and N. Coyle, (eds), *Textbook of Palliative Nursing*. Oxford: Oxford University Press, pp. 767–76.

Randall, F. & Downie, R.S. (2006). *The Philosophy of Palliative Care: Critique and Reconstruction*. Oxford: Oxford University Press.

REFERENCES

Clark, D. (2008) 'History and culture in the rise of palliative care', in S. Payne, J. Seymour and C. Ingleton (eds), *Palliative Care Nursing: Principles and Evidence for Practice*, 2nd edn, Maidenhead: McGraw-Hill/Open University Press, pp. 39–54.

Department of Health (2003) *Building on the Best: Choice, Responsiveness and Equity in the NHS*. London: DH.

Department of Health (2008) *End of Life Care Strategy: Promoting High Quality Care for all Adults at the End of Life*. London: DH.

Hanratty, J. (1989) *Palliative Care of the Terminally Ill*. Oxford: Radcliffe Medical Press.

National Institute for Health and Clinical Excellence (NICE) (2004) *Guidance on Cancer Services: Improving Supportive and Palliative Care for Adults with Cancer*. London: NICE.

Randall, F. & Downie, R.S. (2006) *The Philosophy of Palliative Care: Critique and Reconstruction*. Oxford: Oxford University Press.

Saunders, C. (ed.) (1978) *The Management of Terminal Disease*. London: Edward Arnold.

Speck, P. (ed.) (2006) *Teamwork in Palliative Care: Fulfilling or Frustrating?* Oxford: Oxford University Press.

Sutherland, N. and Stevens, E. (2008) 'Introduction to palliative care', in E. Stevens and J. Edwards (eds), *Palliative Care: Learning in Practice*. Exeter: Reflect Press in Association with the RCN Palliative Nursing Forum, pp.1–40.

Thomas, K. (2003) *Caring for the Dying at Home*. Abingdon: Radcliffe Medical Press.

World Health Organisation (1990) *Cancer Pain Relief and Palliative Care: Report of a WHO Expert Committee*. Geneva: WHO Technical Report Series.

21 information technology

Dion Smyth

DEFINITION

Patient and public participation in healthcare has recently assumed a prominence among professional groups and policy makers in the UK. The increasing emphasis on individual involvement, autonomy and choice is grounded in the various propositions and studies that suggest that empowerment may help people to exercise control over the illness or treatment experience (Cartmell and Coles, 2000; Say et al., 2006). These principles are also enshrined in the various definitions of palliative care (Pastrana et al., 2008). In response to this, participation has been facilitated in numerous ways, including the recognition and use of the internet as a means of providing information, advice and support. This chapter provides an overview of the use of the internet as a healthcare tool.

KEY POINTS

The use of information technology, specifically the internet, for palliative care considers:

- prevalence of internet use;
- relevance of internet use;
- reasons for internet use in healthcare;
- evaluating websites.

DISCUSSION

The last decade has seen an exponential rise in interest in the internet; as a means of communication the availability, applicability, acceptability and widespread accessibility of information on the worldwide web is unparalleled in human history. According to the Office for National Statistics (ONS), in 2008 almost 16 and half million households in the UK (65% of the total) had internet access (ONS, 2008). This represented an increase of 1.23 million over the previous year, and a 46% increase, over 1 million households per year, since 2004. While the home is the most frequent place to access this form of communication technology, the ability to access the internet in the workplace, public libraries, internet cafés or via wi-fi connectivity means that the medium is both popular and pervasive.

According to the ONS data, internet usage is increasing in incidence; overall 69% of adults or 23.5 million people accessed the internet daily. Searching for health-related information is one of the most common internet activities (Eysenbach et al., 2004). Generally, 34% of use, in the UK, focuses on this aspect with at least one-fifth of the 16–24 age groups seeking such material; the frequency rises to a peak of 39% in the 24–44 age groups (ONS, 2008).

The use of electronic health or e-health media, such as worldwide web materials, is therefore likely to contribute to the future management and delivery of healthcare, including palliative care services, requiring professionals to be more technologically aware, literate, competent, and confident. Traditional print-based media have already tacitly espoused an acceptance of the internet, such as publishing web reviews as part of the content, such as 'Web words' within the *International Journal of Palliative Nursing*, or allowing access to full text copy of the academic papers to subscribers, such as via search engines like *Internurse*.

Unlike most conventional services, such as most libraries, the internet provides 24 hour access to an extensive range of information, which may be used to augment conventional care and to confirm the professional advice (Ybarra and Suman, 2006); however, Hesse et al. (2005) found that, overall, almost half of their sample searched online first compared to only 10.9% who would go to the clinician first. Ziebland et al.'s (2004) survey suggested that part of the motivation for patients with cancer using the internet was that it was doubtful their needs would be met through usual healthcare measures. In this study, using the internet allowed the patient to become knowledgeable and competent in their condition and care, and to covertly check up on the acumen of the professional carer without directly compromising the caring relationship. It also allowed them to consider elements of care that may not necessarily form part of mainstream provision, but may often have more of a utility in palliative care, such as complementary and alternative therapies. Ziebland et al.'s (2004) study also reported the role of the internet as a source of social support, where experience of the illness and its treatments could be shared via online narratives. Foster and Roffe (2009) recently described similar benefits of an online forum to self-management of cancer-related problems noting that such an approach allowed patients, with limited conventional means of personal contact, a method of communicating with a broader population of people in similar circumstances.

Using online resources, such as popular search engines for '*Googling*' a diagnosis or details about a treatment need not necessarily be the preserve of patients. Tang and Ng (2006) report how practitioners also need to be proficient with the internet, illustrating how web based searching correctly identified the diagnosis of 15 out of 26 difficult and rare cases, suggesting the usefulness and value of the internet in the therapeutic setting.

Pereira et al.'s (2001) survey of palliative care practitioners found that 88% of participants were searching the internet for clinical information; the majority of respondents also accessed online medical journals or subscription news services; nevertheless, Tieman and Rawlings (2008) found that palliative care nurses' views and utilisation of web-based resources varied according to their role. Specialist nurses were more likely to deem online materials as appropriate for clinical and professional application, which contrasted markedly with registered nurses' more reluctant and reserved attitudes and behaviour. As the internet becomes ubiquitous, and the literature and other medical resources more readily available in this format – comprehensive, relevant, imaginative and inclusive – the professional palliative care practitioners' understanding of how to search and critique the material presented to them will need to develop. In one study, approximately a third of healthcare professionals reported interactions with an internet-informed patient (Podichetty et al., 2006). Keeping abreast of clinical evidence and best practice is a professional responsibility and moral obligation; however, helping patients to discern the quality of what they download and digest may be a new experience for many staff.

Many searches of the internet are incomplete, restrictive and produce less than desirable results. Clauson et al.'s (2008) topical study identified that Wikipedia was able to accurately answer fewer drug information questions than the Medscape Drug Reference; nonetheless, Wikipedia is often one of the first 10 sites listed on search engines such as Google. The hazards of depending solely and uncritically on a publicly edited web site are perhaps most famously found in its use in producing an erroneous obituary for the composer Ronnie Hazlehurst in many of the UK news papers and services (more of which can be read at: www.cnn.com/2007/TECH/11/02/perils. wikipedia/). Thus, for palliative care practitioners as for all professionals, ensuring the reliability and accuracy of the information is paramount.

PRACTICAL APPLICATION OF THE CONCEPT

Jane Smith is a 65-year-old lady, recently diagnosed with Chronic Myeloid Leukaemia. The presence of co-morbidities and absence of an appropriate matched bone marrow stem cell donor means she is unsuitable for a potentially curative transplant; her disease is therefore incurable and she is referred to palliative care services for support. Her treatment is Imatinib (Glivec ®), which is controlling the disease and maintaining her quality of life. She reveals that she has been feeling 'slightly low' since the diagnosis but is loathe to discuss the matter with her GP and does not want to take antidepressant medication as she is 'already taking enough pills' and has worries about dependence and addiction. She tells you that she is considering taking 'St John's Wort', a herbal remedy, as she has read various articles and online testimonials and an online report from a daily news article that says it is an effective therapy (see, for example, www.mailonsunday.co.uk/health/article-1072414/St-Johns-Wort-plant-effective-Prozac-treating-depression-say-scientists.html). She asks you what you think. You are unfamiliar with the treatment but advise her to consider the following points:

- Is the information accurate? For example, what evidence is there for St John's Wort and depression? Has she checked the data against other resources?
- Who is the author of the site(s) she has consulted, can you tell from the web address (such as a personal name, commercial company [.com], government agency [.gov] or non-profit organisation [.org]). Is the author a recognised expert or authority on the subject? Are they stating fact or opinion? Are sources of information stated, and therefore open to verification, such as reference to a refereed or reviewed paper in a recognised, reputable publication? Is there evidence of potential bias, such as site sponsorship or other mercantile concerns such as advertising?
- Is the information source presenting contemporary findings? Is there evidence that the currency of the site, and therefore its content, is up to date? (see www.lib.umd.edu/guides/evaluate.html – Additional details about how to appraise internet material may be found in the 'Further reading' section below).

You search the internet with Jane, and visit a reputable cancer charity, renowned for the quality and clarity of its information – Macmillan Cancer Support (www.macmillan.org.uk/Cancerinformation/QAs/546.aspx) which provides guidance that the herb can 'interact and interfere' with the metabolism of certain drugs, including chemotherapeutic agents. This is cross-referenced against the Merck manual, a well-respected online health library for professionals (www.merck.com/mmpe/lexicomp/imatinib.html) and a search of www.medscape.com which provides consistent and contemporaneous scientific evidence based content reiterating the risk of interaction between the two agents.

CONCLUSION

McMullan (2006) notes that patients are no longer passive beneficiaries of health care, they are clued-up consumers of health information so, rather than feel imperilled by the intelligence the patient brings, she advocates a collaborative approach where patient and professional analyse the content and clinicians act as expert advisors, directing patients to trustworthy health information websites.

Palliative and supportive care aims to assist patients and their family, to adapt to their condition and its treatment of it, through all stages of the journey or illness trajectory and into bereavement. Practitioners help the patient to exploit the benefits of treatment and to experience life, living as well as possible, until death; to do this in an era where imaginative and innovative information technology is continually evolving will increasingly require them to be internet savvy.

See also: *the globalisation of palliative care*

FURTHER READING

Rather than provide further books or journal articles to read, this section provides links to sites that will aid the provision of best practice in utilising the internet in palliative care practice.

www.intute.ac.uk/cgi-in/search.pl?term1=palliative+care&limit=0&subject=All
This is the web address of the palliative care pages of *Intute*, a site that provides free access to web-based educational and research resources that has been selected and evaluated by a network of subject specialists. Typing 'evaluating websites' in the 'search' section opens to 'Internet detective' (also accessible directly at www.vts.intute.ac.uk/detective/), which is an engaging, interactive tutorial about how to critically evaluate internet information.

www.support4learning.org.uk/reference/evaluating_web_sites information.cfm
The support for learning site acts as a 'signpost' to a significant number of resources and organisations that, in this case aid in the process of evaluating websites. Within the section 'Health' may be found two particularly useful sites; firstly the DISCERN criteria, which will be invaluable for any practitioner considering writing any text, whether that is printed or published on the 'net'. The second, is 'Health on the Net', which gives an example of one of, and arguably the most consistent, codes of conduct/accreditation criteria for improving the quality of information on the internet.

www.phru.nhs.uk/Pages/PHD/resources.htm

As clinical evidence becomes more readily available, and easily downloaded from the internet, practitioners will need to be more able at evaluating the data presented to them. The Critical Appraisal Skills Programme (CASP) has helped to expand an evidence-based approach in health and social care, and provides free tools to help with the process of reading and interpreting research articles, helping them to apply knowledge into practice.

REFERENCES

Cartmell, R. and Coles, A. (2000) 'Informed choice in cancer pain: empowering the patient', *British Journal of Community Nursing*, 5(11): 560–4.

Clauson, K.A., Polen, H.H., Kamel Boulos, M.N., et al. (2008) 'Scope, completeness and accuracy of drug information in Wikipedia', *Annals of Pharmacotherapy*, 42(12): 1814–21.

Eysenbach, G., Powell, J., Englesakis, M. et al. (2004) 'Health-related virtual communities and electronic support groups: systematic review of the effects of online peer to peer interactions', *British Medical Journal*, 328: 1166.

Foster, C. and Roffe, L. (2009) 'An exploration of the internet as a self-management resource', *Journal of Research in Nursing*, 14(1): 13–24.

Hesse, B.W., Nelson, D.E., Kreps, G.L. et al. (2005) 'Trust and sources of health information: the impact of the Internet and its implications for health care providers: findings from the first Health Information National Trends Survey', *Archives of Internal Medicine*, 165: 2618–24.

McMullan, M. (2006) 'Patients using the Internet to obtain health information: how this affects the patient–health professional relationship', *Patient Education and Counselling*, 63(1–2): 24–8.

Office of National Statistics (2008) *Internet Access 2008: Households and Individuals*. Available at www.statistics.gov.uk/pdfdir/iahi0808.pdf, accessed 31 March 2009.

Pastrana, T., Jünger, S., Ostgathe, C., et al. (2008) 'A matter of definition: key elements identified in a discourse analysis of definitions of palliative care', *Palliative Medicine*, 22: 222–32.

Pereira, J., Bruera, E. and Quan, H. (2001) 'Palliative care on the net: an online survey of health care professionals', *Journal of Palliative Care*, 17(1): 41–5.

Podichetty, V.K., Booher, J., Whitfield, M., et al. (2006) 'Assessment of internet use and effects among healthcare professionals: a cross sectional survey', *Postgraduate Medical Journal*, 82: 274–9.

Say, R., Murtagh, M., and Thomson, R. (2006) 'Patients' preference for involvement in medical decision making: a narrative review', *Patient Education and Counselling*, 60: 102–14.

Tang, H., and Ng, J.H.K. (2006) 'Googling for a diagnosis – use of Google as a diagnostic aid: internet based study', *British Medical Journal*, 333: 1143–5.

Tieman, J., and Rawlings, D. (2008) 'Exploring nurses' attitudes to, and use of, an online palliative care resource', *International Journal of Palliative Nursing*, 14(12): 587–94.

Ybarra, M.L. and Suman, M. (2006) 'Help-seeking behaviour and the internet: a national survey', *International Journal of Medical Informatics*, 75(1): 29–41.

Ziebland, S., Chapple, A., Dumelow, C., Evans, J., Prinjha, S. and Rozmovits, L. (2004) 'How the internet affects patients' experience of cancer: a qualitative study', *British Medical Journal*, 328: 564. doi:10.1136/bmj.328.7439.564

22 legal and ethical issues in palliative care

Barbara Beard

DEFINITION

Ethics and the law are key components of clinical decision-making in all healthcare settings. An ethico-legal issue can arise when there is conflict between what the patient wants to happen, what Health Care Professionals (HCPs) are able to offer and when there is discrepancy in relation to published guidelines, policy or the law. For example, a person requesting assisted suicide or a person choosing to die at home, against the wishes of their carer.

KEY POINTS

The key points associated with the concept are:

- identification and acknowledgement of the concerns of the patient, carer and professionals;
- knowledge and application of current guidelines and legal requirements;
- facilitation of multi-disciplinary team working, including the patient and/ or carer;
- use of an ethical framework to guide decision-making;
- staying within the parameter of the law;
- sharing the rationale for decisions made with those concerned and offering support for those who may not agree with decisions.

DISCUSSION

Ethical and legal issues arise in everyday clinical situations. While these are primarily managed within the multi-disciplinary team, when there is a particularly difficult issue, the views of a local clinical ethics committee or legal advice may need to be sought. Ethics is not a concept in isolation, but rather part of a holistic approach which includes staying within the law, professional codes of conduct and effective communication with all parties involved. Ethical literature identifies several different approaches to guide ethical decision making.

Ethical frameworks

Normative ethics attempts to answer the question 'what action guides are worthy of moral acceptance and for what reasons' (Beauchamp and Childress, 2008). However, it is well to note that ethical theory does not provide answers, but rather assists in guiding thinking to structure the decision making process when addressing ethico-legal issues. The four principle approach developed by Beauchamp and Childress is one that has been long accepted within health care as identified by the recent publication of the 6th edition of their book on the subject (Beauchamp and Childress, 2008).

Although there are critics of this approach, it is straightforward and is considered more 'direct and action-guiding' than other approaches (Baines, 2008: 141). The principle approach is based on the application of four ethical principles to a specific issue where the four principles would apply except when there is a conflict between two or more of these principles. This then creates an ethical and, sometimes legal, dilemma where a choice has to be made as to which principle applies under those particular circumstances and whether it is within the law.

Application of four ethical principles

The first of these principles is respect for autonomy, the ability for persons to think, understand and make their own decisions without undue influence, whilst also respecting the autonomy of others. Gillon calls this principle the 'first among equals' (Gillon, 2003: 310) as it is increasingly recognised in health care. However, while a person's autonomy has to be respected from an ethical and legal perspective with a refusal of treatment, HCPs are not obliged to permit, for example, a request for assisted suicide or euthanasia, as this would impinge on their own autonomy as well as being outside the law and professional codes of conduct. In addition, the Mental Capacity Act (Department of Constitutional Affairs, 2005) serves to further clarify the right to make an advance decision to refuse treatment (ADRT) for when capacity has been lost and also to guide professionals in how to act when a person no longer has capacity, to ensure that as far as is possible, their wishes are respected.

In contrast, an advance care planning document (Royal College of Physicians, 2009) would enable patients to identify what treatment and care they would prefer to receive, although there is no legal obligation to provide medical care that is clinically inappropriate. An advance care plan may indicate preferences, for example, who a person would like to be present at their death, so facilitating choice and respecting autonomy. Knowledge and application of these and other guidance serve to enhance the decision-making process and subsequently enhance the care of an individual patient.

The second principle, beneficence, is the moral obligation to act for the benefit of another person or in their best interests. Again, the Mental Capacity Act (Department of Constitutional Affairs, 2005) provides guidance on this difficult area as to the responsibilities of a HCP when a person no longer has mental capacity. Closely related to beneficence is the third ethical principle of non-maleficence, which is the duty 'not to inflict evil or harm' (Beauchamp and Childress, 2008: 150). For example, a treatment such as continuing with chemotherapy, when there is no identified potential benefit, may actually be causing more harm to a patient than would its discontinuance if the side effects were a greater burden than the effects of the treatment.

Related to non-maleficence is the principle of double effect, which is the process of relieving symptoms for a patient which may, as a secondary effect, shorten life, although this is not intended. This principle has been used in the past to justify the unintentional shortening of a patient's life in the management of a particular symptom, for example, pain. However, it is largely considered not to be relevant in current clinical practice (Forbes and Huxtable, 2006: 395) due to the developments in effective palliative care, particularly symptom management. The fourth principle, justice, is the ethical obligation to act in a fair way when there are competing claims. For example, justice would not have been served if a patient was not offered effective end of life care in relation to pain relief.

Communication and teamworking

Addressing ethico-legal issues in individual situations requires effective communication with the parties concerned, to actually identify what the issues are from the patient's or family's perspective. It may sometimes be that a patient or the team makes a decision that the family may have difficulty addressing. This may be because of their beliefs that a specific treatment may be of benefit to the patient, even though the patient chooses to refuse it or the team considers is not in the patient's best interests. An example of this could be the decision to withdraw or withhold artificial or clinically assisted hydration that is considered to be in the patient's best interests even though the family may wish the treatment to be continued. Sensitive discussion with the family will be required to explain the situation and offer appropriate support to those who may be finding it difficult to acknowledge the fact that the person they care about is actually dying. Campbell and Partridge (2007) offer guidance in addressing such issues.

It is also important that HCPs do not feel isolated when involved with ethico-legal issues and that the decisions are made within multi-disciplinary team working. Virtue ethics recognises that emotions are an integral part of moral decision making. As Gardiner states: rather than being difficult to control responses, emotions are 'sensitivities that inform our judgements' (2003: 298). As such, it is important that these emotions are acknowledged and worked with when ethico-legal issues arise and that staff feel supported by the team whether they agree with the decision that has been made or not. However, it is also essential that a HCP's beliefs are not forced onto a patient's family as this would be breaching professional codes of conduct.

PRACTICAL APPLICATION OF THE CONCEPT

Ethico-legal issues and effective communication are integral components of clinical practice and cannot be separated from everyday working. For example, on first sight it could be thought that there was an ethical and legal dilemma if a patient requests a professional to assist him to die. However, on further exploration the patient may be wishing to speak about their fears of dying or that they find a particular symptom very distressing, but has not declared this previously. It may be possible to address or reduce any fears and/ or implement effective symptom management by using effective communication. This way, the person's autonomy is respected and the principles of beneficence, non-maleficence and justice can be applied.

Conversely, the person concerned may still feel that they wish their life to be shortened, in spite of all the options above being offered. As this would be contrary to the law, the patient's autonomy could not be respected in this instance although it is essential that the team continues to explore the patient's concerns, support the person as far as they are able and to act in their best interests, offering support to all concerned. Finally, according to Twycross & Wilcock (2001: 2), decision-making in palliative care is based on 'striving to preserve life, but when the burdens of life sustaining treatment outweigh potential benefits, withdrawing or withholding such treatments and providing comfort in dying' are appropriate. A working knowledge of the ethical and legal issues involved will guide this process to the benefit of all concerned.

See also: *communication; good death; multi-disciplinary team; patient choices and preferences; symptom management*

FURTHER READING

Beauchamp, T.L., and Childress, J.F. (2008) *Principles of Biomedical Ethics*, 6th edn. Oxford: Oxford University Press.
Department of Constitutional Affairs (2007) *Mental Capacity Act 2005. Code of Practice.* London: TSO.
Ethox Centre (2009) Available at: www.ethox.org.uk/, accessed 1 April 2009.

REFERENCES

Baines, P. (2008) 'Medical ethics for children: applying the four principles to paediatrics', *Journal of Medical Ethics*, 34: 141–5.
Beauchamp, T.L. and Childress, J.F. (2008) *Principles of Biomedical Ethics*, 6th edn. Oxford: Oxford University Press.
Campbell, C. and Partridge, R. (2007) *Artificial Nutrition and Hydration: Guidance in End of Life Care for Adults.* London: National Council for Palliative Care.
Department for Constitutional Affairs (2005) *Mental Capacity Act.* London: Department of Constitutional Affairs.
Forbes, K. and Huxtable, R. (2006) 'Editorial: Clarifying the data on double effect', *Palliative Medicine*, 20: 395–6.

Gardiner, P. (2003) 'A virtue ethics approach to moral dilemmas in medicine', *Journal of Medical Ethics*, 29: 297–302.

Gillon, R. (2003) 'Ethics needs principles – four can encompass the rest – and respect for autonomy should be "first among equals"', *Journal of Medical Ethics*, 29: 307–12.

Royal College of Physicians (2009) *Advance Care Planning: National Guidelines Number 12.* London: Royal College of Physicians.

Twycross, R. and Wilcock, A. (2001) *Symptom Management in Advanced Cancer*, 5th edn. Oxford: Radcliffe Medical Press.

23 loss, grief and bereavement

Jan Woodhouse

DEFINITIONS

The concept of loss and its link to grief and bereavement have been the central concern of many studies over the last couple of centuries. During our lifetime we experience many kinds of losses such as losing an object, being a victim of theft, loss of innocence, changes to our body through puberty or pregnancy. This chapter focuses on these concepts in relation to palliative care, rather than loss through death, by accidents or acts of violence. Loss, grief and bereavement rightly have separate definitions, as each is a concept in its own right. Waldrop (2007: 197) gives definitions for all three concepts and defines loss in two dimensions; the first is that of physical loss, which is 'when something tangible becomes unavailable'; the second is psychosocial loss, where there is a change in social interactions. As the symptoms of an illness or disease commence, so do the losses and they continue beyond the death of the patient. The response to the losses is grief, which Waldrop (2007: 198) states, citing Stroebe, Hanson, Stroebe and Schut's (2001) definition, is 'a multifaceted response to death and losses of all kinds, including emotional (affective), psychological (cognitive and behavioural), social and physical reactions', whilst Sanders et al. (2008: 497) cite Rando's (2000) definition that it is 'the reaction to the perception of loss'. Bereavement is defined as 'the state of having lost a significant person to death' (Waldrop, 2007: 198) and is a time that can bring a range of emotional responses (Metzger and Gray, 2008).

- Loss is multi-factorial and starts early in the disease process.
- There are physical and psychological aspects of grief and bereavement.
- There are indicators of complicated grief.
- Strategies to acknowledge grief may be useful.

DISCUSSION

Theories of grief

The works of Freud, Bowlby, Worden and Parkes are seminal in postulating theories of loss, grief and bereavement (Bachelor, 2007; Sanders et al., 2008; Tomarken et al. 2008). Freud first termed the word griefwork, and Worden expanded on this by stating that the person suffering loss has certain tasks that they must work through, namely accepting the reality of the loss, working through to the pain of grief, adjusting to the new environment, emotionally adjusting to the new situation and moving on (Bachelor, 2007). Bowlby noted that we encounter grief and bereavement due to attachment and that the stronger the attachment the stronger the sense of loss and grief (Sanders et al., 2008). Parkes's study on grief postulates that the grieving process includes making sense of the loss, challenging or modifying assumptions about the individual's world view (previously based on personal belief systems), and fitting the loss into a general pattern (Bachelor, 2007).

Loss

Turning to the concepts of loss, grief and bereavement in palliative care, the notion of loss can start early on in a disease process. Stuifbergen et al. (2008) note that individuals with chronic conditions, such as multiple sclerosis, talk of having to accept a loss of function. Waldrop (2007) notes that carers of individuals with Alzheimer's often face a protracted 'goodbye', especially when the progress of the disease causes a loss of personality and functional faculties. Sanders et al. (2008) also comment that Alzheimer's causes multiple losses such as socialization, intimacy, roles and responsibilities, and communication and use the term 'ambiguous loss', where the care recipient is physically present but psychologically absent. These aspects may also be present in those with other life-limiting diseases. Metzger and Gray (2008) expand on the loss of communication between partners, by stating that prior to death there may be anxieties and fears about death (and the subsequent consequences), and that these are infrequently discussed. As the patient's health declines, then institutional care may follow and Newson (2008: 321) talks of 'relocation stress', relocation being 'a care option when acute or chronic illness brings about drastic changes in the individual's ability to manage the daily activity of living'. Snowdon and Fleming (2008) focus on residents in nursing homes who experience loss of opportunities and abilities to take part in activities, resulting in sadness and, possibly, depression.

During this time of illness the carer or relative will experience multiple responses. Sanders et al. (2008) identify emotional reactions such as: stress, denial, anger, frustration, a sense of 'burden', and sadness (directed towards what the disease is doing to the patient) at the early and middle stages of the disease progression. Waldrop (2007) comments on the notion of 'distress' felt by carers and uses the National Comprehensive Cancer Network's (2003) definition that states distress is 'An unpleasant emotional experience of a psychological (cognitive, behavioural, emotional), social, and/or spiritual nature that may interfere with the ability to cope effectively with cancer, its physical symptoms, and its treatment.' Distress is further exacerbated by the impact of the physical aspect of being a carer; sleep is disrupted, exacerbation may emerge of pre-existing illness, and carers suffer from physical strain. In the dying phase the emotional responses continue, with anticipatory grief, for example, tearfulness at imagining life without the patient; sadness; longing; loneliness; resignation; and protectionism, for example, focusing on happier moments in life, coming to the fore (Waldrop, 2007; Metzger and Gray, 2008; Sanders et al., 2008).

Bereavement

With this level of emotional turmoil encountered it is not surprising that potential health problems may occur, when the carer and/or relatives enter the grief and bereavement stages, which bring yet more challenges for them. The physiological and psychological symptoms of grief provide an extensive list; the bereaved may suffer insomnia or sleep disturbance, fatigue, loss of appetite, musculo-skeletal aches and pains, increased use of drugs and alcohol, raised blood pressure, increase in smoking, and a susceptibility to illness and disease (Waldrop, 2007; Kowalski and Bondmass, 2008). At the psychological level the bereaved may encounter a lowering of self-esteem; feelings of help-lessness, hopelessness, and unreality; have problems with their memory and concentration; feel despair, anxiety, anger, loneliness; experience a yearning for the past, or regret, or guilt; and will often feel isolated even when amongst families and friends (Waldrop, 2007; Sanders et al., 2008). There may be a preoccupation with thoughts of the deceased and at times the bereaved may be agitated, crying, or withdrawn and may express that they feel unable to cope with life's stresses any more. It is important to note here that these 'symptoms', which tend to medicalize grief, are a normal reaction to an adverse event – in this case, death (Metzger and Gray, 2008). It is normal for the bereaved to oscillate between thoughts of loss and its consequences and then to focus on the everyday practicalities, in an attempt to restore life to normal – this has becomes known as the dual-process model (Stroebe and Schut, 1999, cited in Metzger and Gray, 2008).

If, in this see-saw of thoughts, the bereaved seems to be more in one aspect than another then this may be a sign of maladaptive grieving, or complicated grieving, which may need attention by healthcare professionals. Sanders et al., (2008) make a distinction about what they term as 'separation distress' where the individual is yearning, experiencing illusions and searching for the deceased, which is all part of loss, and that of depression, where the bereaved have a negative interpretation of themselves and/or the world. Metzger and Gray (2008) identify bereavement depression as the bereaved exhibiting a sad mood, apathy, guilt, anxiety, irritability, nervousness and restlessness.

Complicated grief

The notion of complicated grief has many of the aspects previously mentioned such as yearning, crying, and preoccupation with thoughts of the deceased but there may also be disbelief or non-acceptance of the death, longing for the deceased to be as they were before they had the illness, feeling of life being empty, bitterness about the illness, and recurrent images of the lost person, which endure for more than six months and impair the day-to-day functioning of the bereaved (Tomarken et al., 2008; Boelen and Hoijtink, 2009).

Tomarken et al. (2008) suggest that a pessimistic view of the world exhibited by the carer or relative pre-death may lead to complicated grief. Wijngaards-de Meij et al. (2008) also consider how control over the dying phase by the carers (specifically parents of young children and adolescents) impacts on complicated grief. They suggest that being present at the bedside, being able to say goodbye – either before, at the moment of death, or symbolically (poems, planting a tree) – and having direct care of the body may reduce complicated grieving. However, as this was a Dutch study, there may be cultural differences in aftercare of the body.

Triggers and strategies to acknowledge grief

It is recognised that grief can be triggered at any time through items such as photographs, particular music, geographical locations, family events and special occasions, for example, Christmas or other religious feasts, birthdays, general anniversaries and anniversary of the death (Bachelor 2007; Wijngaards-de Meij et al., 2008). These triggers can also serve to acknowledge grief. Weshenfelder (2007) makes the point that healthcare professionals may also need time to grieve and mentions that similar strategies used by the bereaved may help. Strategies might include making a personal memorial, such as having a photo or a memento of the person, writing a journal or piece of poetry, listening to music, and talking with a trusted person – where fears, frustrations, guilt and grief can be aired. These all help to have a continuing bond with the deceased, as it is now recognised that grief and grieving do not end at the funeral or at the first anniversary of the death but continue, often diminishing after two years but may increase again after five years (Kowalski and Bondmass, 2008). Healthcare professionals, who are delivering palliative care, should be mindful that part of the grieving process may be a scrutiny of the care that the deceased received (Sanders et al., 2008) and that an under-standing of loss, grief and bereavement can help to provide support to both the patient and the carer at this critical life event.

PRACTICAL APPLICATION OF THE CONCEPT

Mike was 59 when he was diagnosed with lung cancer. He had divorced from his wife in the previous year, after 25 years of marriage, during which time he had fathered three children. After the divorce he had moved back to the area he had known as a child and acquired a new girlfriend. The eldest son moved in with Mike and took on the role of main carer. At the funeral the ex-wife was upset at not being part of the leading cortege. The girlfriend gained prominence by organising the service sheets and reading out a poem. Several months later the eldest son was experiencing depression and the ex-wife talked of feeling guilty at allowing her marriage to founder. A couple of years after Mike died, all his children were in stable relationships, his ex-wife had remarried and they all spoke of the happier times that were in the past. They could also be moved to tears when thinking of their loss.

See also: *environment of care*

FURTHER READING

Dickenson, D., Johnson, M. and Katz, J.S. (2000) *Death, Dying and Bereavement*. Milton Keynes: Open University/Sage Publications.
Humphrey,G. and Zimpfer, D.G. (2008) *Counselling for Grief and Bereavement*, 2nd edn. London: Sage Publications.
Mallon, B. (2008) *Dying, Death and Grief*. London: Sage Publications.

REFERENCES

Bachelor, P. (2007) 'Practical bereavement', *Health Sociology Review*, 16: 405–14.
Boelen, P.A. and Hoijtink, H. (2009) 'An item response theory analysis of a measure of complicated grief', *Death Studies*, 33: 101–29.
Kowalski, S.D. and Bondmass, M.D. (2008) 'Physiological and psychological symptoms of grief in widows', *Research in Nursing & Health*, 31: 23–30.
Metzger, P.L. and Gray, M.J. (2008) 'End-of-life communication and adjustment: pre-loss com-munication as a predictor of bereavement-related outcomes', *Death Studies*, 32: 301–25.
National Comprehensive Cancer Network (2003) *Distress Management*. Available at: www.nccn.org.professionals/physician_gls/PDF/distress.pdf accessed 4 January 2004.
Newson, P. (2008) 'Relocation to a care home, part one: exploring reactions', *Nursing and Residential Care*, 10(7): 321–24.
Sanders, S., Ott, C.H., Kelber, S.T. and Noonan, P. (2008) 'The experience of high levels of grief in caregivers with Alzheimer's disease and related dementia', *Death Studies*, 32: 495–523.
Snowdon, J. and Fleming, R. (2008) 'Recognising depression in residential facilities: an Australian challenge', *International Journal of Geriatric Psychiatry*, 23: 295–300.
Stuifbergen, A., Becker, H., Blozis, S. and Beal, C. (2008) 'Conceptualization and develop-ment of the acceptance of chronic health conditions scale', *Issues in Mental Health Nursing*, 29: 101–14.

loss, grief and bereavement

Tomarken, A., Holland, J., Schacter, S., Vanderwerker, L., Zuckerman, E., Nelson, C., Coups, E., Ramirez, P.M. and Prigerson, H. (2008) 'Factors of complicated grief pre-death in caregivers of cancer patients', *Psycho-Oncology*, 17: 105–11.

Waldrop, D.P. (2007) 'Caregiver grief in terminal illness and bereavement: a mixed-methods study', *Health & Social Work*, 32(3): 197–206.

Weshenfelder, C. (2007) 'Coping with mortality', *Nursing Home Magazine*, September, 80–4.

Wijngaards-de Meij, L., Stroebe, M., Stroebe, W., Schut, H., Van Den Bout, J.V.D., Van der Heijden, P.G.M. and Dijkstra, I. (2008) 'The impact of circumstances surrounding the death of a child on parent's grief', *Death Studies*, 32(3): 237–52.

24 marginalised groups

Elizabeth Mason-Whitehead

DEFINITION

Since earliest times, marginalised groups have been a constant reminder that the social world that we have created is made up of both 'outsiders' and 'insiders'. Many of us for a variety of reasons such as financial status, mental health or sexual orientation will at some time in our lives have personal experience of being part of a marginalised group. When people find themselves in a position where they require palliative care then their marginalised status becomes more acute and overpowering.

KEY POINTS

- People belonging to marginalised groups are frequently socially excluded from mainstream society, such examples are migrant workers, who may have difficulty with language and find their 'new' culture difficult to understand.
- Marginalised groups often find it difficult to express their views and subsequently their 'voice' is not heard. These may be people who have a learning disability.
- Attracting funding to pursue research that strives to find out more about certain marginalised conditions can be difficult.

- Some marginalised groups are at particular risk of being exposed to poverty.
- Palliative care is not always available to people living in communities who suffer extreme hardship and poverty.
- People from marginalised groups may experience considerable stress and ill health associated with their circumstances, life-style or disability.

DISCUSSION

Over 50 million people die each year, many of whom do not have access to adequate pain control or palliative care (Paice et al., 2008: 173). Estimating how many of these individuals belong to marginalised groups is impossible to know, but the literature and anecdotal evidence suggests that a significant number will be excluded form mainstream society. We are, however, in a position to consider who the marginalised groups are and why they are treated as the 'outsiders' of any given community and no one described this better than Lucy Grealy in her unforgettable account of living with terminal cancer of her jaw (Grealy, 1994).

We could argue that our efforts to try and make sense of our fellow human beings is an unfulfilled journey lasting from the 'cradle to the grave' and an early disappointment is that people's lives are in every sense unequal. Children quickly identify the boy in the class who is 'different' because he has a cleft palate or the little girl who wears the same dress to each party and brings a present that looks woefully inadequate when compared to the offerings of famous brand toys. The trajectory for these children is all too readily associated with an attribute that is seen as 'discreditable' (Goffman, 1963). Their status within their peer group is reduced and their experiences are that of being bullied and excluded has resonance with every generation. For those of us wishing to understand more about marginalised groups we often begin with reading *Stigma: Notes on the Management of Spoiled Identity* by Erving Goffman (1963). Despite its age, this seminal text provides the platform for which any subsequent analysis of marginalised groups begins.

In our identification of a marginalised group, we can refer to the work of Green (2009), who in her analysis of the stigma trajectory has identified some characteristics of what constitutes a marginalised group. By converting these features and others into questions we can begin to understand if a particular group is marginalised. Consider for a moment a patient or client that you have recently cared for, and that caused you concern because they were in some way 'different' and perhaps were trying to cope with more than their long-term condition. By using the Guide in Figure 24:1 you will have some indication of whether they belong to a marginalised group or not. Of course this is not a definitive list, but it is intended to channel and support your concerns.

The starting point for identifying a marginalised group is by understanding the culture to which the group belongs. A 'devalued' group in one culture may be 'revered' in another and this is true of our older population. For example, in India, the Government introduced The Maintenance and Welfare of Parents

1. Is the group *'labelled'* for being *different* in a way that is *negative?*

2. Is the group *stereotyped* in a *disapproving* manner?

3. Is the group *separated* from other members of their community in a way that makes them one of *'them'* as opposed to one of *'us'*?

4. Is the group perceived as having a *'low status'* and being *'inferior'*?

5. Is the group *discriminated* against through *legislation* or *local policy?*

6. Is the group *disempowered* and *stigmatised?*

7. Is the group *socially excluded?*

Figure 24.1   *Guide to Identification of Marginalised Groups*

and Senior Citizens Bill 2006, which made it compulsory for adult children to look after their older parents. The punishment for not doing so is a fine of 500 rupees or three months in jail. By contrast, the American psychologist Todd Nelson has commented extensively on the stereotyping and prejudice against older people in Western societies (Nelson, 2005). Whatever culture we belong to, it is part of the make up of the 'human condition' to separate and compartmentalise people into groups and these are often known as *primitive categories.*

Researching marginalised groups can be difficult. Examples include those people who have a rare condition such as a genetic anomaly and the numbers involved are small or more commonly, where the condition is not regarded as high profile enough such as the elderly. Additionally, funding is difficult to obtain to research 'hard to reach' groups such as prisoners, where access and ethical permission can be challenging.

Poverty is frequently associated with marginalised groups and this may be connected with a number of factors such as a person's ability to earn a salary or actually suffering unemployment, or not finding suitable work because of illness or disability. Some marginalised groups are rejected because their 'condition' is stigmatising, such an example might be a young woman who wishes to work in the beauty industry but despite having the qualifications is repeatedly turned down. The obvious birth mark on her face leads her to believe that this is the cause of her rejection – could she be right?

Access to palliative care is not always available. For example, an asylum seeker with a long-term illness moving from one country to another may feel 'fortunate' to have shelter, food and water. There are now many travelling families in the UK and other countries and they have little access to health services. At this point in time, little is known about their palliative care needs. But clearly in such extreme circumstances the experience of palliative care is something that these marginalised people may not be familiar with.

Let us think about the community where we live and work in and using a simple diagram like the one opposite, to write in those groups of people we

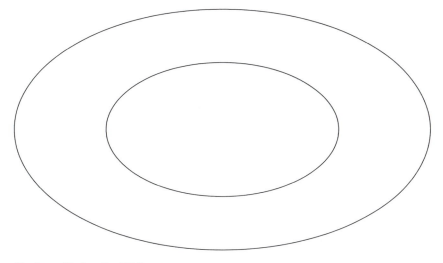

The Inner Circle = the 'IN' Group
The Outer Circle = the 'OUT' (or marginalised) Group

Figure 24.2   *Marginalised Groups Observed in the Communities where we Live and Work*

consider to be the marginalised (or 'out') group and those we believe are seen as the 'in' group. We may be surprised by how these groups differ throughout the country. If we go to Chapter 41, Stigma, we can understand further why we chose our categories and how marginalised groups do not always remain the 'out' group but change with society's expectations and norms, see Figure 24.2.

The bringing together of people from marginalised groups who also require palliative care is undoubtedly one of the most intense tasks faced by both service users and providers. Critically, the challenge begins in developing our understanding of both these experiences and the potential devastating impact when marginalisation and palliative care come together. The way forward is through demonstrating a considerable amount of understanding based upon empathy, knowledge and a genuine desire to be agents for change.

PRACTICAL APPLICATION OF THE CONCEPT

Jenny Wong is a much respected business woman, living in the heart of the Chinese community of a city situated in the north of England. Jenny has maintained her links with the elders of her community and she has noticed that the people who cared for her as a girl are now suffering long-term illnesses and are in much need of help and support themselves. Jenny met with the local Primary Health Care Trust to discuss her concerns about the older people of the Chinese community. A number of meetings were arranged between the local Trust and representatives from the Chinese community and together a care pathway was piloted to deliver appropriate palliative care. The collaboration has been a positive experience for all concerned and provided a platform for further health and social care initiatives. One of the surprising outcomes of this project has been to expel the misunderstandings that the health professionals had of the Chinese community and vice versa. Such an example was Pamela, a health visitor for 20 years, who said she always thought the Chinese community 'always looked after themselves and never wanted us to visit'.

See also: cultural issues; environment of care; palliative care for the person with a learning disability; research; stigma

FURTHER READING

Mason, T., Carlisle, C., Watkins, C. and Whitehead, E. (eds) (2001) *Stigma and Social Exclusion in Healthcare*. London: Routledge.

Nelson, T.D. (2005) *Handbook of Prejudice, Stereotyping and Discrimination*. Hove: Psychology Press.

Young-Breuhel, E. (1998) *The Anatomy of Prejudices*. Cambridge, MA: Harvard University Press.

REFERENCES

Goffman, E. (1963) *Stigma: Notes on the Management of Spoiled Identity*. London: Penguin.

Grealy, L. (1994) *Autobiography of a Face*. New York: HarperCollins.

Green, G. (2009) *The End of Stigma? Changes in the Social Experiences of Long Term Illness*. Abingdon: Routledge.

Nelson, T.D. (2005). *Ageism*. London: Blackwell.

Paice, J.A., Ferrell, B.R., Coyle, N., Coyne, P. and Callaway, M. (2008) 'Global efforts to improve palliative care: the International End-of-Life Nursing Education Consortium Training Programme', *Journal of Advanced Nursing*, 61(2):173–80.

25 multi-disciplinary teams

Moyra A. Baldwin

DEFINITION

In the context of healthcare, a team comprises individuals, in a variety of settings, working together to provide services for patients. Teams combine individuality and inter-dependency; team members, working individually, are accountable for their actions, yet share responsibility and accountability among the team, as they work collectively and collaboratively to meet the team's goals (Mohrman et al., 1995, cited by Borrill et al., 2002; Speck, 2006). Terms relating to teamwork include interdisciplinary, multidisciplinary, and multiprofessional and are often used interchangeably in the literature. Nevertheless there appears to be consensus that a multi-disciplinary team (MDT) involves a range of health and social care professionals, working interdependently, to meet the healthcare needs of patients. While each works independently, MDT members also work collaboratively, together agreeing specific interventions and care management. MDTs are common in medicine, as Speck (2006: 12–13) states, with 'individual members known by their professional identity … . Information within the team is via medical records, each profession adding their contribution to patient care to the record.'

KEY POINTS

- Teamworking is an essential facet of contemporary palliative care.
- Multi-disciplinary teamwork involves individual professionals, generally working independently, communicating and collaborating with other disciplines in the team to plan, agree and implement a gold standard model of palliative care.
- Teamwork requires team skills that enable collective decision-making.

DISCUSSION

Teamwork is a fairly general term that most of us, who are working or have worked in teams, can identify with. Many will have worked together in a variety of ways to care for patients nursed, for example, in hospital settings, their own homes, nursing homes, prisons, or hospices. Some will have worked as generalists and others as specialists within teams, and each will have contributed individually and collaboratively to ensure patients' health and well-being were effectively managed. It is evident that contemporary palliative care embraces multidisciplinary team-working. As noted by Jünger et al. (2007), the number of published articles relating to working in teams bears witness to the fact that teamwork is an essential aspect of palliative care. Since a team comprises two or more people, to function effectively meeting patients' palliative care needs, it is essential that every member shares the goals and philosophy of palliative care. This type of team working, according to Clegg et al. (2008: 92), requires members to be 'psychologically contracted to achieve a common organizational goal in which all individuals involved share at least some level of responsibility and accountability for the outcome'. Since 2004, the time that the National Institute for Clinical Excellence (NICE, 2004) recommended multidisciplinary teamwork for cancer and palliative care services subsequent publications (e.g. Department of Health, 2008) provide the vision and common goal for palliative, end-of-life, care by means of the End-of-Life (EoL) care programme.

The EoL strategy aims to facilitate high quality care for people in the final months of their life. Bélanger and Rodgríguez (2008) evaluated multi-disciplinary work in primary care teams. Reviewing a total of 19 qualitative studies two major areas were highlighted in their analysis, that of organizational strategies and team interactions. In the category of organisational strategies analysis revealed four themes namely: (1) investing time and resources towards team building; (2) developing locally adapted and flexible organizational structures: (3) defining clear roles and communicating effectively; and (4) sharing power and involving all health professionals. These components exist in the End-of-Life care programme (Department of Health, 2008), time and resources have been invested in England to disseminate three key tools: Gold Standards Framework (GSF), Liverpool Care Pathway and Preferred Place (priorities) of Care. In addition, other locally developed tools have been incorporated demonstrating the flexibility of organisational structures.

In respect of the third theme, defining clear roles and communicating effectively, NICE (2004: 7) guidance recommends:

> Each multidisciplinary team or service should implement processes to ensure effective inter-professional communication within teams and between them and other service providers with whom the patient has contact. Mechanisms should be developed to promote continuity of care, which might include the nomination of a person to take on the role of 'key worker' for individual patients.

The key worker aspect is of particular importance in securing palliative care for vulnerable and disenfranchised populations e.g. prisoners or people with concurrent mental illness. Mahmood-Yousuf et al. (2008), using a qualitative interview-based case study approach, explored the impact of the GSF on relationships and communication in primary palliative care teams that had implemented the GSF in the previous two years. Analysis of general practitioners', district nurses' and specialist nurses' responses indicated improvements in both communication and teamwork, and consequently 'benefits for terminally ill patients'. The study also provides evidence of sharing power and involving health professionals as the multidisciplinary team meetings were valued 'transforming administratively-focused events … into opportunities for discussing patients and consolidating relationships between GPs, district nurses and Macmillan nurses' (Mahmood-Yousuf et al., 2008: 260). The researchers acknowledge that the practices involved in the study were 'early adopters' of the GSF; there were nevertheless some who were more circumspect about the relative strengths of formal MDT meetings.

Policy documents report that healthcare staff need appropriate knowledge, skills and attitudes to work collaboratively and successfully in teams. MDTs are not merely the domain of primary care teams, and as collaborative decisions undertaken within MDT meetings are reported to have significant benefits for patients (Ruhstaller et al., 2006), the MDT is important for the patients with palliative care needs, irrespective of the setting in which care is delivered.

Good communication, clear objectives, openness and confrontation, and appropriate leadership are some of the many qualities Woodcock (1989) considers necessary for teams to work effectively, all of which are essential if patients' needs are to be successfully managed. Ruhstaller et al. (2006) note that national and international studies report improvements in care and treatment outcomes for patients suffering from a variety of conditions as a result of decisions made by multidisciplinary teams. They demonstrate holism in action – a decision made by the whole team is greater than the sum of the decision made by the individual parts (professionals) within the team. Involvement of all members of the team in a single discussion 'is more effective and the joint decision more accurate than the sum of all individual opinions' (Ruhstaller et al., 2006: 2460). Unnecessary interventions are avoided; patients are involved in the decision-making process and are thus rightly engaged, as service users, in the management of their palliative care needs.

The GSF's seven Cs: communication, co-ordination, control of symptoms, continuity, continued learning, carer support, and care in the dying phase have improved healthcare professionals' knowledge and confidence (Oliver, 2003). This programme of multi-disciplinary team-working is enabling anticipatory care, reducing crises and inappropriate admissions: improvements in practice and outcomes as indicated by After Death Analysis (2008).

There is clear evidence of successful teamworking in palliative care but an observation that might be worth noting, if only to avoid complacency, is the result of a survey undertaken in 2007 and reported in the Nursing Standard. While NHS staff claimed they worked in teams, fewer than half considered they worked in effective teams. Effective multi-disciplinary team working in palliative care, as noted above, involves a range of appropriate professionals working collaboratively and interdependently, with the patient and family, to agree decisions and implement planned care. The MDT enhances palliative care services and delivery when it is committed to common goals, respects others and uses effective communication skills.

PRACTICAL APPLICATION OF THE CONCEPT

Ellen, a 54-year-old single lady who lives with her mother, was admitted to the hospice for symptom management. She was admitted for specialised management of uncontrolled pain due to bone metastases, extensive arm lymphoedema and a malodorous fungating right breast. At the MDT meeting Ellen's progress was discussed, pain management and wound care were agreed, and plans for discharge home were in the early stages. Nurses reported that Ellen's pain was being well managed, there were no concerns about polypharmacy, the Clinical Nurse Specialist (CNS) and physiotherapist reported reduction in lymphoedema and Ellen's progress with exercises, and the music therapist reported that Ellen had attended her first session, and would probably attend for more. Ellen's wound was causing her embarrassment due to the offensive smell and the team's decision was to alter the dressings, if no progress was reported by the next meeting they would refer to the tissue viability nurse. Discharge plans included the social worker's specialist input. Ellen lived with an elderly, rather frail mother who also had care needs. The social worker and Ellen agreed that community staff would be involved in her care when she returned home. The social worker also helped with Ellen's finances. This particular meeting demonstrated collaboration and communication: each of the professionals working both independently and interdependently, communication among them enabled a whole team decision regarding Ellen's care while an in-patient as well as future plans for her discharge home to the care of the primary care team employing the GSF.

See also: *agencies; attributes of palliative caring; communication; holism*

FURTHER READING

Payne, M. (2000). *Teamwork in Multiprofessional Care*. Basingstoke: Macmillan.
Speck, P. (ed.) (2006) *Teamwork in Palliative Care: Fulfilling or Frustrating?* Oxford: Oxford University Press.

REFERENCES

After Death Analysis (2008) Briefing paper: The After Death Analysis (ADA) Audit Tool. Available at: www.goldstandardsframework.nhs.uk/content/care_homes/ADA%20 Briefing%20Paper%20July%202008%20FINAL.pdf, accessed 18 January 2009.

Bélanger, E. and Rodgríguez, C. (2008). 'More than the sum of its parts? A qualitative research synthesis on multi-disciplinary primary care teams', *Journal of Interprofessional Care*, 22(6): 587–97.

Borrill, C., West, M., Dawson, J., Shapiro, D., Rees, A., Richards, A., Garrod, S., Carletta, J. and Carter, A. (2002) *Team Working and Effectiveness in Health Care*. Aston Centre for Health Service Organisation Research, Birmingham. Available at: http://homepages.inf.ed.ac.uk/jeanc/DH-glossy-brochure.pdf accessed 9 September 2009.

Clegg, S., Kornberger, M. and Pitsis, T. (2008) *Managing and Organizations*, 2nd edn. London: Sage.

Department of Health (2008) *End of Life Care Strategy: Promoting High Quality care for all Adults at the End of Life*. London: DH.

Jünger, S., Pestinger, M., Elsner, F., Krumm, N. and Radbruch, L. (2007) 'Criteria for successful multiprofessional cooperation in palliative care teams', *Palliative Medicine*, 21(4): 347–54.

Mahmood-Yousuf, K., Munday, D., King, N. and Dale, J. (2008) 'Interprofessional relationships and communication in primary palliative care: impact of the Gold Standards Framework', *British Journal of General Practice*, 58(549): 256–63.

National Institute for Clinical Excellence (NICE) (2004) *Guidance on Cancer Services: Improving Supportive and Palliative Care for Adults with Cancer*. London: NICE.

Nursing Standard (2007) News. *Nursing Standard*, 21: 28. p.11.

Oliver, G. (2003) 'Times are changing', *Cancer Nursing Practice*, 2(5): 15–17.

Ruhstaller, T., Roe, H., Thürlimann, B. and Nicoll, J. (2006) 'The multidisciplinary meeting: an indispensable aid to communication between different specialities', *European Journal of Cancer*, 42: 2459–62.

Speck, P. (2006) 'Team or group – spot the difference', in P. Speck (ed.), *Teamwork in Palliative Care: Fulfilling or Frustrating?* Oxford: Oxford University Press, pp. 7–24.

Woodcock, M. (1989) *Team Development Manual*. London: Gower.

26 organ donation

Natalie A. Pattison

DEFINITION

Organ donation is an umbrella term for donation of tissues and/or organs from one person to another. Donation can be from a person who has died, often referred to as cadaverous donation, or from a living donor. This chapter deals with organ donation from a person who has died.

KEY POINTS

Areas that are addressed are:

- Organ donation is a background issue.
- Physiological, legal and consent issues determine what can be donated and who can donate.
- There are specific issues relating to heart-beating donors.
- Practicalities of donation: include practice and emotional issues.
- Nursing considerations in organ donation require sensitivity.

organ donation

121

DISCUSSION

Background to organ donation and transplantation

Organ donation is an emotive issue. It can be construed as something positive to come out of a tragedy of a person dying (Beasley et al., 1997) but raises many legal, ethical, moral and emotional issues. This chapter will outline some of the aspects to consider when thinking about organ donation. The first transplant, using a kidney, was carried out in the 1950s and transplantation medicine has grown hugely since then. This chapter is primarily concerned with organ donation from people who have died.

What can be donated? Physiological issues

The term organ donation now also includes tissue donation and includes:

- kidneys,
- heart (including valves*),
- lungs,
- liver,
- pancreas,
- small bowel.

These organs all have to be donated immediately or, very rarely and only for kidneys, within one hour of death.

*Heart valves can be transplanted within 72 hours. Transplant teams need to be contacted at the earliest opportunity, before death where possible, to ensure the organs are viable.

Other tissues transplanted include:

- skin,
- trachea/larynx,
- corneas,
- brain,
- bone.

These organs can generally be donated within 24–36 hours, depending on which organ. More recently, faces and hands have been transplanted but this is a new development and, as such, is not yet common practice.

Limitations

There are certain limitations to donation. HIV and CJD mean donation is proscribed from these people. However, certain infectious diseases such as Hepatitis B, metastatic malignancy, other prion diseases, and Alzheimer's may also be barriers to donating but this can be discussed with a transplant team. Scarring of organs may also mean that they cannot be donated. There are clear reasons for strict limitations. In the case of metastatic disease in cancer, the metastatic process could lead to donation and transplantation of diseased tissue or organs. Blood is taken and tested from all potential donors. Doing this rules out issues such as HIV and hepatitis. Families are made aware that this procedure is required.

Who can donate? Legal and consent issues

The Human Tissue Act (HTA) (HMSO, 2004) has led to several implications for those wishing to donate. Adults without capacity and children are able to donate organs. Adults without capacity can donate if the circumstances for donation are compliant with Mental Capacity Act and Human Tissue Authority (HTA) regulations (HMSO, 2006). In the case of adults without capacity it would be the clinical teams, the HTA and any family members who decide about organ donation. It could be argued that family members and transplant or clinical teams could potentially have a conflict of interest and may not be sufficiently independent. An independent assessor may be required. Children would had to have expressed a wish that they wanted to donate and be deemed legally competent to do so, or parents and legal guardians can also donate their child's organs if the child's wishes were unknown (UK Transplant, 2009).

In the case of a person who has died, the wishes of the deceased donor, who has consented to organ donation while capacitous, *should* take precedence. Registering on the NHS Organ Donor Register is considered as consent for organ donation. The register (Section 15 of Code 2) provides guidance as to how clinicians should deal with situations in which relatives object to donation. It is stated that families do not have the legal right to veto or overrule the deceased's wishes. This is difficult to manage in clinical practice since some perceive clinicians to have a duty of care to the family too, but ultimately it could be argued that the person's wishes take priority. However, if the wishes of people who have died are unknown then trained health professionals should sensitively provide enough information to facilitate a decision. If wishes are unknown and a person had previously been nominated to deal with the use of their body after death (a nominated representative), they can give consent to donation. Once a decision has been made, it must be respected (HTA, 2009).

The future of organ donation lies in presumed consent (Department of Health, 2008). Unless stated otherwise, everyone will be presumed to have given consent for organ donation. In other words, organ donation might become an opt-out, rather than opt-in, system.

Heart-beating donors vs non heart-beating donors

In many situations, such as heart transplantation and those outlined earlier, it is better to donate from a person whose heart is still beating. Heart-beating donors have suffered a brain stem death and their organs are kept perfused and functioning by ventilation and sometimes by cardiac measures, such as inotropes and cardiac bypass, until brain stem tests have been carried out. Once these tests have verified brain stem death status, these people are *legally dead*. There is no legal definition for death but the Department of Health (1998) guidelines suggest that a definition of death should be regarded as 'irreversible loss of the capacity for consciousness, combined with irreversible loss of the capacity to breathe' (Department of Health, 1998: 7).

Brain stem death, however, presents a big challenge for families who have to come to terms with the fact that their loved one still feels warm, still has a heart beat, and is breathing with the aid of a ventilator. Nurses and medical staff have to introduce the idea that while the person appears alive, they have no capacity for consciousness and have, in fact, died. Testing for brain stem death in the UK follows the Department of Health (1998) Code of Practice and must be carried out by a registered medical practitioner who is not a member of the transplant team (UK Transplant, 2009). This is to avoid any potential accusations of conflict of interest. Brain stem death testing in the UK involves a series of clinical tests carried out by two practitioners. Patients have to fulfil certain criteria before brain stem death testing can be considered, and these can be found on the Department of Health website (see reference list).

Practicalities of donation: practice and emotional issues

Transplant teams have a wide role supporting potential recipients, helping nurse patients after brain stem death ready for transplantation operations, dealing with bereaved families and ensuring organs reach their intended destination. In sudden death in emergency situations some departments will administer preservative medication to allow for a potential option of kidney donation. This provides a very small window of time until wishes can be ascertained.

If there is any doubt as to a person's eligibility for donation, the transplant coordinator should be informed. The earlier the transplant team is involved, the greater the chance of successful donation and the more support the team can give to both staff and families.

Organ donation can lead to family conflict and is an emotive subject which should be approached carefully (Wilkinson, 2007). However, this should in no way deter conversations about donation with families of eligible people. People donate, or ask for their family member's organs to be donated, for a number of reasons, including altruism, feeling that something positive has come out of tragedy, giving meaning to death (particularly when untimely and sudden) and personal philosophies on donation.

Nursing considerations in organ donation

Nurses should have the confidence to sensitively and gently approach the issue of organ donation with families. This should be part of a whole team approach where doctors and other team members agree that donation would be clinically appropriate. Previous wishes can be carefully explored to find out what the person who has died would have wanted if they had not expressly outlined their wishes with a donation card, for example. Nurses should consider organ donation issues when the person is dying, where possible, and prior to administering care after the person has died: last offices.

Summary practice considerations

- Having the courage to raise the issue of organ donation.
- Preparing the family (and person who has died, where appropriate – in liaison with transplant team) for organ donation.
- Raising awareness in your place of practice for patients or clients, staff and families.
- Informing the organ donation team, in a timely manner, that the person wishes to donate organs.

PRACTICAL APPLICATION OF THE CONCEPT

An organ donation card, signed two weeks previously, was seen among the personal effects of a 35-year-old breast cancer patient who was dying on the ward. When she had died, her husband said that he did not wish for her to donate organs. The nurse on the ward was under the impression that because she had cancer she could not donate and therefore did not pursue this with her husband.

Brief exploration of issues and some questions to reflect on:

The nurse could have contacted the organ donation teams who would have outlined that as a cancer patient, she might potentially have been able to donate her corneas, depending on her metastases. Why did the husband not wish to donate? Were his reasons being sensitively and carefully explored? She had expressly wished for her organs to be donated. What does this mean ethically and morally?

See also: *coronial process; death; legal and ethical issues; loss, grief and bereavement*

FURTHER READING

www.dh.gov.uk/en/Healthcare/Secondarycare/Transplantation/index.htm
www.bts.org.uk
www.uktransplant.org.uk

REFERENCES

Beasley, C., Capossela, C., Brigham, L., Gunderson, S., Weber, P., and Gortmaker, S.L. (1997) 'The impact of a comprehensive, hospital-focused intervention to increase organ donation', *Journal Transplant Coordination*, 7: 6–13.

Department of Health (1998) *A Code of Practice for the Diagnosis of Brain Stem Death*. London: Department of Health. Available at: www.dh.gov.uk/en/Publicationsandstatistics/ Publications/PublicationsPolicyAndGuidance/DH_4009696, accessed 10 March 2009.

Department of Health (2008) *Organs for Transplants: A Report from the Organ Donation Taskforce*. London: Department of Health.

HMSO (2004) *Human Tissue Act*. Available at: www.opsi.gov.uk/ACTS/acts2004/ ukpga_20040030_en_1, accessed 19 March 2009.

HMSO (2006) *The Human Tissue Act 2004 (Persons who Lack Capacity to Consent and Transplants) Regulations 2006*. Available at: www.opsi.gov.uk/si/si2006/20061659.htm, accessed 19 March 2009.

Human Tissue Authority (HTA) (2009) *Code of Practice 2: Donation of Solid Organs for Transplantation*. London: Department of Health. Available at http://www.hta.gov.uk/legislationpoliciesandcodesofpractice/codesofpractice/code2donationoforgans.cfm?faArea1=customwidgets.content_view_1&cit_id=669 accessed 10 September 2010

UK Transplant (2009) www.uktransplant.org.uk.

Wilkinson, T.M. (2007) 'Individual and family decisions about organ donation', *Journal of Applied Philosophy*, 24: 26–40.

27 organisational management of palliative care

Steve Kirk

DEFINITION

The word 'organisation' comes from the Greek word 'organon' which means tool or instrument. Organisational management is not really a distinct concept within business and management and in fact all the adjective does is distinguish it from the management of things that are not organisations. Therefore, one potential definition is the running of an entire organisation to ensure that all elements are coordinated to get the best out of the human resources. The goal of organisational management is to influence employees or groups of employees to act in line with the organisation's strategy.

KEY POINTS

Organisation management of palliative care addresses the following aspects:

- organisational culture;
- difference between voluntary and public sector;

- challenges and opportunities;
- structure and systems;
- leadership and management;
- strategic and operational decisions;
- organisational performance;
- people and management;
- the customer!

DISCUSSION

What is organisational management?

All organisations are made up of people, as the essential component, and then structures and systems that enable people to function as effectively as they can and help the organisation in delivering its purpose and philosophy – or its vision/mission statement. However, once people start working together, they often develop relationships and hierarchies that contribute to the development of cultures that can influence an organisation's development either positively or negatively. Any management structure should facilitate the best ways of influencing that culture for the positive benefit of the organisation. The leader, either at the top or in the subsections throughout the organisation, needs to have well-developed skills in harnessing the abilities, skills and attitudes of the individuals to enable them to function as efficiently as they can, in order to contribute to the organisation's purpose.

In addition, structures and systems around communication, engagement, involvement and education, learning and development all need to interrelate to ensure the competence of the individual and the organisation. The development of a strategy enables the organisation to focus where it wants to go, that is, the destination. An annual planning process that maps out the part of the journey the organisation or business needs to complete en route to the destination helps everyone to understand and contribute to that route.

Finally, the organisation needs systems and structures to manage problems that might pop up on the way, such as capability, competence, capacity, coping, comments and complaints, in addition to knowing how well the organisation is doing against the targets it sets itself, such as performance indicators, quality standards or outcome measures.

organisational management

127

HOW FAR DO GENERAL ISSUES ABOUT ORGANISATIONAL MANAGEMENT APPLY TO PALLIATIVE CARE?

Culture

Understanding the relevant culture is critical to understanding the techniques that might be used to influence that culture. If it is an open and understanding culture that accepts new ideas easily and embraces change willingly, the task of influencing that culture should be easier than in one that is static, resistant to change and finds innovations difficult and threatening.

There are many writings on organisational culture but one of the best is Handy's (1993) book *Understanding Organisations*. Handy suggests there are differing types of culture that are influenced by the leadership and people in the organisation. He describes these cultures so that people can recognise where they are and develop strategies to manage their way through the change process. Although the culture in NHS palliative care services is often similar to the pervading NHS culture that surrounds it, hospices can often differ dramatically from hospice to hospice. These can vary from those entrenched in the past and on the good work that they do, to ones that have embraced the elements of a modern forward-thinking organisation which looks to see what it needs to do: to ensure it continues to be able to provide its services and adapts to the competing requirements that abound in current society. Schein (2004) also looks at the link between culture and leadership in organisations and helps one to understand how culture influences organisations. The art of influencing the culture, by applying behavioural science knowledge to improve its effectiveness, is called organisational development (Walshe and Smith, 2007).

Strategy

The aim of organisational management is for a manager to influence colleagues to act in line with the organisation's strategy, therefore the set goals need to be built around the achievement of this aim. This would include the development of the strategy, involvement in the strategy, and signing up to the strategy at all levels. This means developing a strategy from the bottom up, through questionnaires, workshops, presentations, visiting all areas, in summary, fully understanding where the issues lie. The development of the strategy should be an organisation-wide document contributed to by all staff and not forgetting external stakeholders. NHS organisations often fall under the hospital-wide strategy and it can be difficult to pull out the specifics of the strategic nature of where the particular palliative care service is heading. Hospices differ significantly as to whether they have a strategy or not. Those that do usually have a clear idea of where they are heading.

Communication

Communication systems are essential to engaging and informing the individuals who work there. These can be informal or formal but, either way, they need to be focused on clarity, connections, cascading, contributions and commitment.

- Clarity – using simple language that all, from the customer (for example, patient, relative, retail, fundraising) to the Trustees, understand and can relate to.

- Connections – ensuring that information is passed through systems that enable all corners of the organisations to be engaged. Written information could include being attached to payslips, sent by e-mail, joining in group meetings, but checks need to be in place to ensure these methods are effective.
- Cascading – ensuring managers have systems in place to ensure information gets through to those difficult parts to reach, often hands-on staff and volunteers.
- Contributions – ensuring that information is not always top down but mostly bottom up, with everyone encouraged to develop the organisation.
- Commitment – a real passion that everyone has a responsibility to pass information on from management through to the individual taking responsibility for reading and digesting information.

Do palliative care settings bring other specific challenges/demands/opportunities in relation to organisational management?

Organisational management in palliative care is no different than in any other type of organisation. However, the type of organisation can influence both positively and negatively the level of difficulty involved, and this is as true of palliative care settings as it is of other organisations. Most palliative care is delivered in NHS settings or in hospices, and these offer different challenges and demands.

NHS palliative care services generally have a mixed component led by the NHS agenda and local demands and priorities. The mix of services usually includes providing some inpatient beds and also a service covering every ward in the hospital. The staff teams are usually quite small and therefore organisational management is usually fairly straight forward, although there may be conflicting lines of responsibility between the organisation of the smaller team/organisation and the needs of the bigger organisation, the hospital, such as in relation to hospital targets or waiting lists.

In contrast, the majority of specialist palliative care is provided by hospices, which are charitable organisations, receiving about one-third of income from the NHS but relying on fundraising to raise two-thirds of all income. This creates extra complexity in terms of organisational management, as the complex mixture of charity law and company law has to be balanced against the demands of the commissioners: the NHS and the demands of a service predominantly funded by charitable donations. This means that factors such as providing support and development to volunteers, complying with Trading Standards, and with the Gambling Commission, make the management of these organisations quite complicated. There are also key issues around Boards of Trustees that need careful handling to ensure the organisation works at its most effective. There are advantages and disadvantages of being either in an NHS palliative care service or in an independently-run charitable hospice.

Nearly three-quarters of the hospice resource in the UK is provided by individual, self-run charities where small boards of trustees usually white, middle-class, male trustees influence the development of the hospice, and the majority of the funding is provided directly by the public through fundraising. The rest is provided by the NHS and by a few larger national charities such as Marie Curie and Sue Ryder Foundation. For the purposes of this chapter, the term staff will include employees and volunteers.

Palliative care is a complex area, in that there is often significant emotional involvement by the staff electing to work in this area and therefore the culture can develop in a very protective and caring, maternal way. One of the key differences between hospices and other organisations is that much of the workforce is voluntary, and this can substantially influence the response to change, weight of opinion on change, and the change process. In situations where the number of volunteers exceeds the number of paid staff, effecting changes in the organisation can bring particular challenges in terms of consultation, communication, and involvement. Managers rely on the goodwill of volunteers and, therefore, can often be reluctant to face the same issues they would have with paid staff in the same way, particularly around performance issues. Issues can often be left unresolved, fearing volunteers might be upset. Volunteers may also feel they have a right to criticise the organisation in a way that paid staff would not, which can be either very positive or negative depending on how this is managed.

What has your experience of running hospices led you to believe/value in terms of organisational management?

Organisational management is closely related to management of performance. Performance management supports organisations in realising their plans by improving their management through the process of planning, monitoring and adjusting plans. This also enables the staff (and volunteers) within the organisation to act within the boundaries of the organisational strategy.

Performance management improves the management of an organisation by coordinating management reporting, strategy development and review, and organisational and process management. Performance management improves the overall management of an organisation when it ensures management information is available to those that need it, and creates conditions within the organisation for staff to reflect the organisational strategy.

Organisational management can be focused on three areas which need management and coordination, namely strategic, tactical and operational fields. Strategic management focuses on the vision and strategic objectives are developed, while tactical management concentrates on the application of tasks, functions and procedures. Operational management provides guidance and working arrangements through the development and sharing of good day-to-day policies and procedures, operations manuals and guidance. In addition, systems for management reporting, control and the provision of management information are critical.

PRACTICAL APPLICATION OF THE CONCEPT

I worked in three hospices, and none of these had a strategy in place when I commenced. In some respects having no strategy is like starting a journey without a destination. You will end up going somewhere but it may not be where you would have liked. In addition, having no map or route to the destination means you may end up taking either twice as long or going out of your way to get there. If you want the scenic route that's fine, especially if that's what your plan is, but if your plan is to get there as quickly as possible, then this route would not work for you. Therefore, a formal, or even informal, business plan is essential in order to enable all your colleagues to contribute and know what is happening.

Having worked both in a hospice run by a national charity and two independent hospices, each of which had never had a strategy in place, I would suggest that it is not uncommon for charitable hospices not to have developed a long-term plan. The development of the strategy was the first task I undertook in each hospice, engaging and involving people from all areas. The development of good communication systems, a good organisational structure and putting consistent systems in place was the framework that enabled the hospices to identify their key purposes, celebrate their successes, and identify targets that would help them to develop their future services for the benefit of patients, staff and the whole hospice community.

See also: *finance issues and the organisation of palliative care; multi-disciplinary teams*

FURTHER READING

Handy, C.B. (1993) *Understanding Organisations*, 4th edn. New York: Oxford University Press.

REFERENCES

Handy, C.B. (1993) *Understanding Organisations*, 4th edn. New York: Oxford University Press.

Schein, E.H. (2004) *Organisational Culture and Leadership*, 3rd edn. San Francisco, CA: Jossey-Bass.

Walshe, K. and Smith J. (2007) *Healthcare Management*. Maidenhead: Open University Press, pp. 342–55.

organisational management

131

28 palliative care and the person with cancer

Debbie Wyatt

DEFINITION

Palliative care forms one element of cancer care for those individuals who have advanced disease. The general principles of palliative care apply to this particular client group, but there are a number of palliative care issues specific to people with cancer or those caring for them. This chapter will therefore focus on the relationship between palliative care and the person with cancer.

KEY POINTS

- Cancer care has a high national profile.
- Palliative care is an aspect of cancer care for those individuals who have progressive disease.
- There is a misconception that cancer is always synonymous with death and dying.
- Although palliative care provision has tended to focus on those with advanced cancer, there is a drive to widen the availability of quality palliative care to all adults at the end of life.
- It is important to have knowledge and understanding of specific cancer-related issues in palliative care.
- The multi-professional approach to palliative care in cancer is advocated.

DISCUSSION

The context of cancer and palliative care

The national profile of cancer has risen since cancer was identified as one of five key target areas for improving the health of the population of England (Department of Health, 1992). The subsequent Policy for Commissioning Cancer Services (Expert Advisory Group on Cancer, Department of Health, 1995) made recommendations for improving cancer services in England and

Wales and made specific recommendations for improving palliative care in cancer, including the need for multi-disciplinary palliative care teams containing specialists in palliative care. Subsequent Department of Health and Scottish Executive cancer strategies have demonstrated the Government's commitment to the investment and reform of cancer services and within that, a commitment to investment in specialist and supportive palliative care (Department of Health, 2000, 2007a; Scottish Executive, 2001). The National Institute for Clinical Excellence (2004) also produced cancer specific palliative care guidance in 'Improving Supportive and Palliative Care for Adults with Cancer'. While more recent documents such as the End of Life Care Strategy (Department of Health, 2008) promote high quality palliative care for all adults at the end of life, the provision of palliative care services has for some years focused primarily on the needs of people with advanced cancer. This is evidenced, for example, by the high ratio of people with advanced cancer compared to those with non-cancer-related diseases who are cared for in hospices. Although the principles of palliative care are relevant to people with any life-limiting illness, caring for people with advanced cancer may require additional knowledge, understanding and skills specific to their disease and treatments. It is important to dispel the misconception however, that all people with cancer have a life-limiting illness.

Concept of palliative care and its application to cancer

Cancer and palliative care are sometimes referred to synonymously, with an assumption that a cancer diagnosis will always lead to pain and death. The media's negative depictions of cancer reinforce this association and research suggests that negative attitudes also exist among health care professionals as well as the general public (Kearney et al., 2003). Although more than 1 in 3 people will develop cancer in their lifetime, cancer survival continues to improve and end of life care forms only part of cancer care for those people who go on to develop advanced disease.

While not all people with a cancer diagnosis require palliative care, healthcare professionals working in a range of general and specialist settings require knowledge and understanding of the specific needs of people with life-limiting cancers in order to recognise problems early, intervene where appropriate to reduce loss of function and ill-health and to promote quality of life. This may include knowledge of potential symptoms associated with advanced cancer, therapeutic interventions and the prevention of cancer treatment-related problems. If symptoms resulting from a spinal cord compression are not recognised and treated early, for example, the patient may suffer permanent loss of motor function. Similarly, the effects of hypercalcaemia can lead to the misery of nausea and can also hasten death. Interventions to manage specific symptoms include breathlessness management for lung cancer and compression bandaging for lymphoedema. An understanding of treatment-related problems include the prevention and management of constipation in patients receiving opioids, and of nausea and vomiting in patients receiving particular emetogenic chemotherapy. Knowledge of the psychological impact of a cancer diagnosis on individuals and their families is also well recognised and this is reflected in the requirement for senior healthcare professionals working predominantly with people with cancer to undertake advanced communication skills training to enable them to more effectively support patients through their cancer diagnosis, treatments and palliative care (Department of Health, 2007b). An understanding of the specific needs of people with cancer is therefore an important aspect of cancer palliative care, but knowledge of cancer care and management can also inform other aspects of palliative care practice.

Multi-professional approach to cancer and palliative care

The multi-professional approach to cancer and palliative care has been advocated for a number of years (Department of Health, 1995, 2000, 2007a) and sits comfortably within the current drive for multiprofessional collaboration in health care (Department of Health, 2007b). Medical, nursing and allied health professionals (AHP) are represented at national and local cancer network level to guide good practice in cancer care and management, but knowledge of the roles of different members of the multiprofessional team and the part they can play in contributing to quality cancer care is key to promoting appropriate communication between practitioners. Rehabilitation, for example, plays an important role in cancer and palliative care and may involve a range of healthcare professionals such as nurses, physiotherapists, art therapists, speech and language therapists and occupational therapists. Appropriate referral is dependent upon adequate referral mechanisms and an understanding of how interventions can enhance the patient experience. Some professions have their own special interest groups and/or guidelines which inform and help to develop cancer and palliative care practice such as the Royal College of Nursing, Chartered Society of Physiotherapy, College of Occupational Therapists, British Dietetics Association and Society and College of Radiographers. This reinforces the important role of the multi-professional team in cancer palliative care in both hospital and community settings.

PRACTICAL APPLICATION OF THE CONCEPT

Joe, a 58-year-old man who had undergone surgery five years ago for bowel cancer, was admitted to a general medical ward with weakness and altered sensation in both legs. Nursing staff immediately advised him to lie flat in bed and following medical assessment, he was referred to diagnostic imaging for an MRI scan which revealed a spinal cord compression. He was referred to a clinical oncologist who prescribed radiotherapy to the spinal lesion and the hospital palliative care team were alerted. The palliative care specialist nurse discussed the cause of Joe's symptoms with him in the presence of his wife at his request. Referrals were made to the occupational therapist, physiotherapist, and dietician for assessment and rehabilitation which culminated in Joe's return home with the support of Community GP, Nursing, Physiotherapy and OT services. Home adaptations were recommended and facilitated. Joe's symptoms improved markedly for a period of weeks and he enjoyed this period of independence including a weekly visit to a local day hospice. He was aware of his prognosis, however, and was able to discuss with his wife and Community Macmillan nurse, his preference to stay at home should his condition deteriorate. When Joe's condition suddenly deteriorated, a Community package was organised, including commencement on the Liverpool Care of the Dying pathway and Hospice at Home interventions. Joe died in comfort in his own home and his wife continued to be supported in the following weeks through hospice bereavement support.

Relevance to practice

- Early recognition of symptoms of spinal cord compression and subsequent treatment minimised further damage to spinal cord and maximised quality of life for as long as possible.
- Effective communication skills were required to discuss prognosis, discuss preferred priorities of care and handle difficult emotions.
- Knowledge of the roles of other members of the multi-professional team led to appropriate referrals in both hospital and community settings which maximised the patient's independence and quality of life.
- Patient and family involvement were facilitated effectively through knowledge of key reports and effective communication skills.

See also: *communication; organisational management of palliative care; policy drivers; rehabilitation in palliative care; stigma*

FURTHER READING

College of Occupational Therapists, *HOPC (HIV/AIDS, Oncology & Palliative Care)*. Available at: www.cot.org.uk/Homepage/Specialist-Sections/COTSS__HIV-AIDS,_ Oncology_and Palliative_Care, accessed 16 June 2009.

The Chartered Society of Physiotherapy (2003) 'The role of physiotherapy for people with cancer', available at: www.csp.org.uk, accessed 16 June 2009.

Royal College of Nursing (2003) *A Framework for Adult Cancer Nursing*. London: RCN.

palliative care and the person with cancer

REFERENCES

Department of Health (1992) *The Health of the Nation*. London: The Stationery Office.

Department of Health (1995) *Policy for Commissioning Cancer Services: Report of the Expert Advisory Group on Cancer*. London: The Stationery Office.

Department of Health (2000) *NHS Cancer Plan*. London: The Stationery Office.

Department of Health (2007a) *Cancer Reform Strategy*. London: The Stationery Office.

Department of Health (2007b) Creating an Interprofessional Workforce: An Education and Training Framework for Health and Social Care. London: The Stationery Office.

Department of Health (2008) *End of Life Care Strategy*. London: The Stationery Office.

Kearney, N., Miller, M., Paul, J., Smith, K. and Rice, A. M. (2003) 'Oncology health care professionals' attitudes to cancer: a professional concern', *Annals of Oncology*, 14: 57–61.

National Institute for Clinical Excellence (2004) *Supportive and Palliative Care for Adults with Cancer*. London: NICE.

Scottish Executive (2001) *Cancer in Scotland: Action for Change*. Edinburgh: Scottish Executive.

29 palliative care for the person with a learning disability

Sue Read

DEFINITION

People with a learning disability are described as having a reduced ability to understand new or complex information, or to learn new skills (impaired intelligence) with a reduced ability to cope independently (impaired social functioning) which started before adulthood and with a lasting effect on development (Department of Health, 2001). This definition, therefore, describes a whole range of people who may present with a variety of differing abilities, personalities, characteristics and needs. The help that individuals need may vary over time and indeed throughout their lives, and particularly when a diagnosis of a life-limiting condition is made. There is a slowly developing evidence base around the challenges that people with a learning disability often present to generic palliative care services and professionals together with recommendations as to how palliative care services can be more accessible to people who have a learning disability.

KEY POINTS

- Marginalised groups may struggle to access palliative care and support.
- Recognising ill health in people with a learning disability may be difficult.
- Collaborative working is the key to effective care and support.

DISCUSSION

Palliative care and support should be available to anyone diagnosed with a life-limiting condition, yet it is recognised that the social context in which the person lives may affect both where that person dies and the access to the range of services that are needed as the person approaches the end of their life (Oliviere and Monroe, 2004). Death never occurs in a vacuum but within a social context, and factors such as poverty, social class, age, ethnicity, religion and disability, usually influence how and when people die (Oliviere and Monroe, 2004). Marginalised groups in particular, for example people with learning disabilities, may struggle to access palliative care and support at the time they need it most, for a whole host of reasons.

Health and health needs

People with a learning disability are identified as being one of the most socially excluded groups in Britain today (Department of Health, 2001), particularly when it involves health care. At least 2.5% of the population have a learning disability in the United Kingdom, yet they still remain one of the most marginalised groups in contemporary society (DH, 2001), particularly when it comes to death and dying. They are recognised as having poorer health than the general population and face particular barriers when they come to be in need of palliative care and support. Inherent social problems including unemployment, limited exercise and restricted social activities, obesity, poor diet and additional health problems such as increased incidence of epilepsy and dementia all serve to compound the general health status of people with learning disabilities (Mencap, 2004).

Ill health and persistent challenges to effective support

People with a learning disability are generally living longer, and are affected by the same diseases as the rest of the population. However, they are reported to have a lower incidence of bronchus, prostate and breast cancer, but a significantly higher incidence of gastro-intestinal cancer (58% compared to 25% of general population) (Hogg et al., 2001). There is also 20–30 fold greater risk of leukaemia in people with Down's syndrome among this population (Hogg et al., 2001). People with a learning disability often have unmet health needs, and reportedly die of illnesses that are potentially curable (Mencap, 2007). Actually meeting the health needs of people with a learning disability may be difficult because some people with a learning disability may not be able to:

- differentiate between personal good-health and ill-health;
- recognise potential (and actual) health problems;
- communicate in a way that is meaningful to others who do not know them;
- identify and describe symptoms of change in health status in a meaningful way;
- understand difficult concepts such as death, dying or palliative care;
- ask for referrals to clinics for health screening;
- assert their health needs and wants in clear, understandable ways.

Similarly, some health professional carers may:

- not understand what having a learning disability actual means;
- lack knowledge about certain associated conditions (such as cerebral palsy, Down's syndrome);
- assume that all people with learning disabilities cannot communicate/do not have the capacity to consent;
- harbour misguided fears and anxieties about people with learning disabilities;
- be unfamiliar with this population;
- not have received any education/training on supporting people with a learning disability;
- not know who to contact for help and support.

Such inabilities may serve to prevent ill health such as malignant and/or non-malignant diseases from being spotted by others, both personal and professional carers, at an early stage or being treated quickly, efficiently and effectively. This means that some illnesses/diseases are diagnosed late, with poor outcomes. Diagnostic overshadowing, where the learning disability itself is perceived by professional carers to mask any presenting ill-health symptoms, can also lead to illnesses being overlooked and mistaken for other conditions such as the learning disability itself. Professionals may struggle to find the words to explain to a person with a learning disability that their illness is incurable, and that death will ensue, meaning that some individuals may not even know they are dying. When death is kept hidden and secret, and the dying person is socially excluded from the dying process and is deliberately excluded from any decision-making surrounding their impending death, such as funeral arrangements or making a will, this has been described as disenfranchised death (Read, 2006).

Overcoming the barriers

Many people with a learning disability struggle to communicate in an effective way, and reciprocal communication with unfamiliar health professionals may be difficult. It is crucial for palliative care professionals to establish the most meaningful way of communicating with each individual and to talk to the significant people, for example, family members, personal carers, health facilitators, in the person's life to establish what this system might be. Effective communication can involve having a planned approach to care using signs, symbols, pictures, sign language, such as Makaton, and by using clear words and pictures to establish a person's understanding of, for example, disease, treatment options/preferences and preferred place of care.

Everyone has the right to know, and similarly not know, their diagnosis, and decisions about truth telling and avoiding collusion remain important. The person breaking difficult news to a person with a learning disability has to be considered very carefully; preferably someone familiar with the person with a learning disability should be there; in familiar surroundings; using an appropriate communication system such as the ARCH model (Read, 2009).

Assessment is the key to any effective diagnosis and subsequent treatment, and communication is thought to be one of the biggest obstacles to accurate medical assessment (Tuffrey-Wijne, 2003). Assessment tools that may be useful with people with a learning disability are the DisDat tool (Regnard et al., 2003) a tool specifically designed for this population that focuses on distress from an observational perspective over time; and the Abbey Pain Scale, a simple tool designed for people with dementia.

Collaborative working across both learning disability and palliative care services is the key to providing effective palliative care and support for people with learning disabilities. Education and training can be the basis for understanding of both learning disability and palliative care, and shared learning can help to promote effective support.

PRACTICAL APPLICATION OF THE CONCEPT

John had Down's syndrome, and was arriving at the hospice for a short stay to help him to manage his pain and associated symptoms related to his stomach cancer. John had been prepared for this visit by a local health facilitator: a professional who works closely to reduce the barriers between specialist, learning disability services and generic health and palliative care services. John had routinely visited the hospice before, prior to admission, and the health facilitator had taken photographs of the hospice and where it was situated. She also took photographs of John's named nurse who would be taking care of him; the reception area inside the hospice; and the in-patient unit where he would be sleeping. These pictures were then arranged in a folder so that John could be helped to familiarise himself with the hospice prior to his admission. Such a planned approach to his care made it easier for John to understand what was happening to him and where he was going. John brought his camera with him so that he could take more pictures of what was happening to him while in respite.

See also: *communication; marginalised groups; stigma*

FURTHER READING

Blackman, N. and Todd, S. (2005) *Caring for People with Learning Disabilities Who Are Dying*. London: Worth Publishing.

Read, S. (ed.) (2006) *Palliative Care for People with Learning Disability*. London: Quay Books.

Read, S. and Morris, H. (2009) *Living and Dying with Dignity: The Best Practice Guide to End-of-Life-Care for People with a Learning Disability*. London: Mencap.

REFERENCES

Abbey pain scale, available at: http@//stratishealth.org/clientuploads/documnets/NH_EO_PainWebEx_Handout1_011708.pdf, accessed October 2008.

Department of Health (2001) *Valuing People: A New Strategy for Learning Disability for the 21st Century*. London: DH.

Hogg, J., Northfield, J. and Turnbull, J. (2001) *Cancer and People with Learning Disabilities: The Evidence from Published Studies and Experiences from Cancer Services*. Kidderminster: BILD.

Mencap (2004) *Treat Me Right!* London: Mencap.

Mencap (2007) *Death by Indifference*. London: Mencap.

Oliviere, D. and Monroe, B. (2004) *Death, Dying and Social Differences*. Oxford: Oxford University Press.

Read, S. (2006) *Palliative Care for People with Learning Disabilities*. London: Quay Books.

Read, S. (2009). *Living with an Illness that I Will Die From: A Guide for Professional Offering Palliative Care and Support*. Staffordshire: Keele University.

Regnard, C., Matthews, D., Gibson, L., Clarke, C. and Watson, B. (2003). 'Difficulties in identifying distress and its causes in people with severe communication problems', *International Journal of Palliative Nursing*, 9(3): 173–6.

Tuffrey-Wijne, I. (2003) 'The palliative care needs of people with learning disabilities: a literature review', *Palliative Medicine*, 17: 55–62.

key concepts in palliative care

30 palliative care and the person with mental ill-health

Julie Bailey-McHale and Catherine Black

DEFINITION

The focus of this chapter is those people who are living with a severe and enduring mental illness and subsequently develop a physical condition that requires specialist palliative care. Severe and enduring mental illness includes mental health problems such as schizophrenia, bi-polar affective disorder and severe depression (Ellison, 2008). There is some debate within mental health literature regarding whether other illnesses such as depression, anxiety and anorexia should also be included. It could be argued that these traditional descriptions are neither holistic nor individualistic as only the individual can truly articulate the degree of severity of their experiences. However, currently the vast majority of research uses this approach.

McCasland (2007) highlights that people with severe and enduring mental illness have an earlier mortality compared to the general population. Farnam, Zipple, Tyrrell and Chittinanda (1999) estimate that people with mental illness die between 10 and 15 years earlier. Phelan, Stradins and Morrison (2001) suggest that research in many countries consistently confirms that psychiatric patients have high rates of physical illness that go largely undetected.

KEY POINTS

- People with severe and enduring mental illness have a higher risk of developing a life-threatening physical illness compared with the general population.
- People with severe and enduring mental illness and a physical condition requiring specialist palliative care may experience difficulties accessing appropriate care at appropriate locations.
- Both mental health services and palliative care services have skills to provide holistic, integrated care for this group of people but need to work closely together to ensure that all of their complex needs are met successfully.

DISCUSSION

Lack of access to specialist palliative care services

Service users and mental health professionals have for a long time high-lighted the demoralising effects of social exclusion experienced by those with a mental health problem. This exclusion extends to all aspects of life and access to timely and appropriate palliative care treatment is no excep-tion. Koffman and Camps (2008) highlight the difficulties diagnosing physical conditions in people with severe and enduring mental illness. This is due to a number of factors including the unconventional manner of pres-entation of symptoms that may be associated with this group. This impacts upon engagement which can be fraught with difficulties as palliative care staff are faced with behaviours, cognitions and emotions that may seem bizarre or extreme. This can be exacerbated by a potential unwillingness to verbalise pain and willingness to tolerate physical symptoms, such as non-healing lesions, to a greater extent than the general population. Such diffi-culties can lead to late presentation and diagnosis of disease. Late presentation creates difficulties for palliative care specialists to manage symptoms successfully regardless of any co-morbidities. For those with existing severe and enduring mental illness it leads to a unique and complex set of needs. The literature suggests that professionals from both specialities feel uncomfortable and unskilled in managing these complex needs (McCasland, 2007; Ellison, 2008).

Consent and capacity

The issue of capacity and the expression of choice is a crucial aspect for any client group. Capacity can be seen as the ability to comprehend and value information regarding diagnosis and potential prognosis of disease, and to make informed decisions regarding treatment choices. An assump-tion can sometimes be made that those with a diagnosis of a mental health problem usually lack capacity. This is clearly not the case, indeed only a relatively small percentage of people with a mental health problem are assessed as lacking capacity. However, those working in palliative care settings, and indeed any non-mental health setting, may mistakenly assume a lack of capacity in an individual with a mental illness diagnosis. Woods et al. (2008) demonstrated that a presumption of lack of capacity can mean that the person is excluded from conversations about their diagnosis and prognosis, and that such conversations take place with rela-tives. Foti et al. (2005a) demonstrated that this presumption of lack of capacity is incorrect. While those with severe and enduring mental illness may have more difficulties in understanding the information about diagno-sis and prognosis than the general population, they can be supported with appropriate levels of communication and education to make appropriate advance directives.

Advance directives

Within mental health settings the whole notion of advance care directives is now established and there are many examples of service users making advanced decisions regarding the treatment they prefer when unwell. This approach is also well recognised and utilised within palliative care settings (McCasland, 2007). As the notion is familiar within both settings, it is appropriate that it should be used for individuals who require care from both services.

Foti et al., (2005b) found that the majority of mental health service users could engage in advance care planning surrounding end of life issues. They recommend that such discussions should be commenced at the same point as for the general population.

Multi-professional working

Multi-professional working is seen as a key aspect within all areas of health care. Poor inter-professional liaison between mental health practitioners and palliative care practitioners, when caring for people with dual needs, can create a 'loud silence' (McGrath and Holewa, 2004) which can create a barrier to effective assessment, care and management. There would appear to be real fear among practitioners of each other's speciality and client population (McCasland, 2007). This is despite a significant degree of shared knowledge, values and aspirations.

Black et al. (2001) demonstrated the synchronicity between mental health practitioners and palliative care practitioners. They highlighted many similarities including the non-curative aspect of the specialities, the important role in aspects of non-physical care, the vital nature of the client–professional relationship and that the locus of control in both specialities lies with the individual. They identified differences as the use of facilitation and confrontation, and management of physical symptoms. As there are more similarities than differences, care of patients with dual needs should be successfully managed by high-quality collaboration between the teams, staff education and support, symptom control algorithms and a focus on the involvement of and control by the individual concerned.

The leadership of the team should not be fixed but should vary depending on the location of the client's care and the prioritisation of their symptom burden at any given time – but members of the team from both specialities have the skills to lead the care (Ellison, 2008). The use of appropriate care pathways, planning and shared documentation will ensure high quality, appropriate care, to meet the wide-ranging and complex needs of individuals with concurrent severe and enduring mental illness and palliative care needs.

PRACTICAL APPLICATION OF THE CONCEPT

At an unsuccessful MDT meeting two weeks ago, organised to plan her care in relation to her metastatic breast cancer, Sarah became very distressed. The number of people in the room, many of whom Sarah didn't know, overwhelmed her and her voices began to shout at her. Her key worker, whom Sarah had known for many years since her schizophrenia was diagnosed, had asked for the meeting to end.

Since then, two members of the palliative care team have visited Sarah several times on the unit, and on one occasion, her key worker has taken Sarah to visit the hospice. The two specialist teams have met in full to discuss the management of both aspects of Sarah's care – her schizophrenia and her metastatic breast cancer.

At today's meeting, only those who have established a relationship with Sarah are present. All those attending are mindful of the pacing and level of information shared. Sarah is less anxious and so able to manage her voices more effectively, and play a more active role in the decision-making process.

See also: *legal and ethical issues in palliative care; marginalised groups; multidisciplinary teams*

FURTHER READING

Addington-Hall, J. (2000) *Positive Partnerships: Palliative Care for Adults with Severe Mental Health Problems*. London: National Council for Hospice and Specialist Palliative Care Services and Scottish Partnership Agency for Palliative and Cancer Care. Report on occasional paper 17.

Woods, A., Willison, K., Kington, C., and Gavin, A. (2008) 'Palliative care for people with severe persistent mental illness: a review of the literature', *The Canadian Journal of Psychiatry*, 53(11): 725–36.

REFERENCES

Black, C., Hanson, E., Cutcliffe, J. and Goward, P. (2001) 'Palliative care nurses and mental health nurses: sharing common ground?', *International Journal of Palliative Nursing*, 7(1): 17–23.

Ellison, P. (2008) *Mental Health and Palliative Care. Literature Review*. London: Mental Health Foundation.

Farnam, C.R., Zipple, A.M., Tyrrell, W. and Chittinanda, P. (1999) 'Health status risk factors of people with severe and persistent mental illness', *Journal of Psychosocial Nursing*, 7: 16–21.

Foti, M.E., Bartels, S.J., Van Clitters, A.D., Merriman, M.P. and Fletcher, K.E. (2005a) 'End-of-life treatment preferences of persons with serious mental illness', *Psychiatric Services*, 56(5): 585–91.

Foti, M.E., Bartels, S.J., Merriman, M.P., Fletcher, K.E. and Van Clitters, A.D. (2005b) 'Medical advance care planning for persons with serious mental illness', *Psychiatric Services*, 56(5): 576–84.

Koffman, J. and Camps, M. (2008) 'No way in. Including disadvantaged population and patient groups at the end of life', in S. Payne, J. Seymour and C. Ingelton (eds), *Palliative Care Nursing: Principles and Evidence for Practice*, 2nd edn. Maidenhead: Open University Press, pp. 362–82.

McCasland, L.A. (2007) 'Providing hospice and palliative care to the seriously and persistently mentally ill', *Journal of Hospice and Palliative Nursing*, 9(6): 305–13.

McGrath, P. and Holewa, H. (2004) 'Mental health and palliative care: exploring the ideological interface', *International Journal of Psychosocial Rehabilitation*, 9(1): 107–19.

Phelan, M., Stradins, L. and Morrison, S. (2001) 'Physical health of people with severe mental illness', *British Medical Journal*, 322: 443–44.

key concepts in palliative care

Woods, A., Willison, K., Kington, C. and Gavin, A. (2008) 'Palliative care for people with severe persistent mental illness: a review of the literature', *The Canadian Journal of Psychiatry*, 53(11): 725–36.

31 palliative care and the person with a non-cancer diagnosis

Andrea Dean

DEFINITION

At the beginning of the twenty-first century the majority of deaths follow a period of chronic illness such as Coronary Heart Disease (CHD), Motor Neurone Disease (MND), Multiple Sclerosis (MS), Parkinson's Disease (PD), Chronic Obstructive Pulmonary Disease (COPD), or dementia (Department of Health, 2008). Until fairly recently, palliative care was primarily geared towards patients with a cancer diagnosis. However, the Coronary Heart Disease Collaborative (Department of Health, 2004) acknowledges that 'heart failure produces greater suffering and is associated with a worse prognosis than many cancers' and has attempted to define current practices and make recommendations for new services to support heart failure patients and their carers. Considering neurological conditions, there is little empirical evidence to identify the palliative care needs of these patients and their carers and how this can be addressed (Byrne et al., 2009). To create distance from the common association between 'palliative care' and 'cancer care' the term 'end of life care' is quite often used to emphasise the need for support for patients with palliative care needs who have a non-cancer diagnosis.

KEY POINTS

- The dimensions of palliative care are expanding to encompass a broader range of conditions and meet the care needs of changing demographics.

- The trajectory of disease can present challenges regarding palliative/end of life care as the terminal phase of some non-cancer conditions can be difficult to predict.
- Neurological conditions may need care planning for cognitive, behavioural and communication problems.
- Palliative care/end of life care has evolved from care of patients with cancer conditions and although there are some clinical similarities in non-cancer conditions, there are also considerable differences which need to be recognised and planned for.
- Meeting the palliative/end of life care needs for people with non-cancer conditions will require understanding from healthcare staff at all levels.

DISCUSSION

In the past 100 years the demographics of death in relation to age, cause and place of death have changed radically. Many conditions which were once considered terminal are now considered chronic as patients may live for many years from diagnosis. Indeed, with many people now living into their eighties and nineties, it can in fact be quite difficult to define when 'dying' commences and the complex factors that lead to death can only be understood retrospectively (Byrne et al., 2009). Hence, it might even be questioned whether 'generalist palliative care' is an appropriate term as one needs to be diagnosed as dying or at the end of life to qualify for that care. There may be many settings which deliver palliative care although it is not labelled as such, for example, care homes for older people and day centres. This demands the development of broader knowledge and expertise in palliative care.

Although immense progress has been made in the past 50 years in providing palliative care to ameliorate complex and distressing symptoms when curative options have been exhausted, most of this progress has been available to cancer patients. Despite a comparable level of need, there are fewer and less coordinated palliative care services for patients with non-cancer conditions.

People with a non-cancer diagnosis can be especially disadvantaged because of the differences in trajectories of disease. For example, although lung cancer diagnosis might often be perceived as delayed, once the prognosis was made, it is clearly understood. Cardiac failure, on the other hand, can be a chronic illness with episodes of acute deterioration that often necessitate emergency admission to an acute hospital, punctuating an overall progressive decline with the terminal phase being difficult to predict. Heart failure symptoms can be wide-ranging and severe. Symptoms can include anorexia, nausea, constipation, low mood, muscle wasting, dyspnoea due to increased congestion of the blood vessels in the lungs, fatigue due to impaired muscle blood flow and oedema due to fluid retention. Pain is a symptom of severe heart failure although this is not well recognised (Gibbs et al., 2002). Treatment for heart failure can slow the disease, but does not stop its progression. Studies of

Table 31.1 Comparison of experience of patients

Lung cancer	Cardiac failure
Cancer trajectory with clearer terminal phase; able to plan for death	Gradual decline with intermittent episodes of acute deterioration; sudden, usually unexpected death with no distinct terminal phase
Initially well but told you are ill	Feel ill but told you are well
Good understanding of diagnosis and prognosis	Little understanding of diagnosis and prognosis
'How long have I got?'	'I know it won't get any better, but I hope it won't get any worse'
Relatives anxious	Relatives isolated and exhausted
Swinging between hope and despair	Daily grind of hopelessness
Lung cancer takes over life and becomes overriding concern	Much comorbidity; heart often not seen as main issue
Treatment world dominates life, more contact with services and professionals	Shrinking social world dominates life, little contact with health and social services
Feel worse on treatment: coping with side effects	Feel better on treatment: work of balancing and monitoring in the community
Financial benefits accessible	Less benefits with uncertain prognosis
Specialist services often available in the community	Specialist services rarely available in the community
Care prioritised early as 'cancer' and later as 'terminally ill'	Less priority as a 'chronic disease' and less priority later as uncertain if yet 'terminally ill'

Source: Adapted from Murray et al. (2002).

patients have shown that they are often symptomatic, and that their symptoms have a significant impact on their quality and style of life. A holistic approach to care is needed, along with collaboration of members of the multidisciplinary team, as physical symptoms are frequently influenced by social, spiritual and psychological issues. Patients with long-term neurological conditions also have to contend with various forms of disablement and pain, together possibly with cognitive, behavioural and communication problems which makes care delivery and advance planning for care in the last stages of life complex and challenging (Byrne et al., 2009)

Although there are similarities in clinical characteristics between heart disease and cancer, there are considerable differences in care needs and experience of patients (Table 31.1).

Doyle et al. (2005) consider that before palliative care can be considered, one must accept that the patient's condition is terminal, and there are two factors which hinder the palliative care of patients with advanced

147

heart failure. These are the difficulty in predicting decline with physical well-being not being uniformally progressive, and, second, the fact that most patients and health professionals do not view heart failure as a terminal disease despite the mortality seen in the condition. This aligns with some issues for patients with neurological conditions who also can have a longer and more variable disease trajectory, prone to relapse and remission making 'end of life' stage harder to recognise. Murray et al. (2002) found that patients with heart failure had less information about and poorer understanding of their condition and prognosis and were less involved in decision-making. The primary concern of lung cancer patients was facing death, but frustration, progressive losses, social isolation and the stress of a complex medical regime dominated the lives of the heart failure patients. Murray et al. (2002) concluded that end of life care for patients with advanced cardiac failure and other non-cancer diseases should be proactive and designed to suit their specific needs rather than diagnosis. Effective palliative care should be an integrated component of patient care, not merely a care addition at the end stage of disease.

The End of Life Care Strategy (Department of Health, 2008) recognised that to attain quality end of life services it would be necessary to promote a cultural shift in attitude and behaviour within the health and social care work-force. The Department of Health (2009) aimed to achieve this cultural shift by developing competences and core principles and identifying related com-munication skills at all levels within the workforce, although they acknowledge that the work is a 'milestone in development and not a finished product'.

PRACTICAL APPLICATION OF THE CONCEPT

Julia, a 72-year-old patient with end stage heart failure, was admitted to a cardiac ward within a general hospital. She had become very breathless during the night and her husband had called an ambulance. The following day she felt a little better but became increasingly anxious as she felt her condition was deteriorating. In the afternoon she became very breathless, asking the student nurse to sit with her and asking her why this was happening. She was becoming very distressed saying 'Am I going to die? I can't breathe, I don't want to die, I'm not ready please tell me.' The student notified one of the staff nurses who said to check that Julia had her oxygen mask on. Julia's husband and family came in to see her at 2pm. As it was not visiting time they were told to go away and come back later. Minutes after they left Julia arrested and the student nurse called for help. There was confusion as someone asked about next of kin. A health care assistant was sent to the hospital café to look for the relatives. Julia died before her husband and family were found and returned to the ward.

See also: *holism; symptom management: common symptoms; symptom management: difficult/complex symptoms*

Byrne, J., McNamara, P., Seymour, J. and McClinton, P. (eds) (2009) *Palliative Care in Neurological Disease*. London: Radcliffe-Oxford.

Connolly, M. (2000) 'Time for non-cancer', *International Journal of Palliative Nursing*, 6 (2): 91–3.

REFERENCES

Byrne, J., McNamara, P., Seymour, J. and McClinton, P. (eds) (2009) *Palliative Care in Neurological Disease*. London: Radcliffe-Oxford.

Department of Health (2004) *Palliative and Supportive Care for Advanced Heart Failure*. London: The Stationery Office.

Department of Health (2008) *End of Life Care Strategy: Promoting High Quality Care for All Adults at the End of Life*. London: The Stationery Office.

Department of Health (2009) *Common Core Competences and Principles for Health and Social Care Workers Working with Adults at the End of Life*. London: The Stationery Office.

Doyle, D., Hanks, G., Cherny, N. and Calman, K. (eds) (2005) *Oxford Textbook of Palliative Medicine*, 3rd edn. Oxford: Oxford University Press.

Gibbs, J., McCoy, A., Gibbs, L., Rogers, A. and Addington-Hall, J. (2002) 'Living with and dying from heart failure: the role of palliative care', *Heart*, 88 (Suppl.2): 36–9.

Murray, S.A., Boyd, K., Kendal, M., Worth, A., Benton, F. and Clausen, H. (2002) 'Dying of lung cancer or cardiac failure: prospective qualitative interview study of patients and their carers in the community', *British Medical Journal*, 325: 929.

32 palliative care education

Karen Manford-Walley

DEFINITION

Education for palliative care encompasses a myriad of concepts and skills needed to match the diverse nature of care delivery, additionally education is delivered at many levels by a range of providers, and in many settings. These settings may include higher education institutions and specialist palliative care services within hospital and community settings, with delivery to both single professional groups and inter-professional participants. Educational provision may include higher education accredited undergraduate and postgraduate modules and programmes, additionally short courses and study days contribute to the varied education provision (Foyle and Hostad, 2004).

KEY POINTS

Palliative care education encompasses:
- inter-professional education;
- palliative care education to all disciplines;
- public involvement in palliative care education;
- changing educational delivery.

DISCUSSION

Pivotal to the validity and relevance of palliative care education is the ability to respond to the continual development of the knowledge base. Developments in treatment modalities are influencing the management of life-limiting diseases. Additionally, greater knowledge from research regarding genetics, disease development and progression is impacting upon screening, diagnosis and treatment, as well as our understanding of risk factors. Political drivers and government agendas are changing the way that services are organised, funded and delivered. In addition, moral and ethical debates relating to palliative care are receiving more public and political attention.

Educators need to be active in facilitating inter-professional educative strategies to meet the widening professional input evident in palliative care, as no one professional group can provide the complex, physical and psycho-social needs of patients and their families as they make the journey from screening, diagnosis, treatment, palliative care, and the terminal phase of their condition (Richardson, 2004). Added to this is the acknowledgement that educational methods themselves are evolving to encompass differing modes of delivery and development of this knowledge. The didactic, peda-gogical structure of education is not primarily seen as the only method of educational delivery, and other methods, including work-based learning, e-learning, and experiential learning, are important aspects of education. These alternative methods of educational delivery may be seen as the pre-ferred method for accessing educational interventions for busy healthcare providers, where study leave is seen as an optional extra in current economic challenging times.

Consequently, to facilitate palliative care education, that is both contempo-rary and relevant, educators need to be constantly reviewing curriculum, objectives and evaluating educational outcomes. This will serve to achieve validity and balance, both in the integration of academic and practical applica-tion of palliative care education, as well as developing partnerships between educators and professionals to enable students to integrate knowledge and professional learning successfully.

Interactions between healthcare providers and patients may be shaped, in part, by their educational preparation and training, in addition to their lived experiences. Significantly, educational initiatives for cancer and palliative care workers have been encouraged in several documents. Notably the National Institute for Health and Clinical Excellence (NICE) Guidelines in Improving Supportive and Palliative Care for Adults with Cancer (NICE 2004) recommended that all nurses and allied health professionals should have some training in cancer and palliative care, and that it should be taught and assessed appropriately. This document also endorsed inter-professional education, and acknowledged that professionals should be able to recognise patients' needs more effectively, and work collaboratively to improve the care that patients receive.

However Blunden et al. (2001) argue that the educational and training needs in the field of cancer and palliative care are not always addressed. This appears to be significant when considering the educational needs of health care support workers, who may often feel unprepared and ill-equipped to care for people with cancer and their relatives. Banks-Howe et al. (2003) high-lighted that health care support workers' skills will come under close scrutiny, especially as this group of staff may need to develop skills and knowledge to undertake duties that may have been previously performed by registered nurses. Waldron et al. (2008) suggest one strategy to introduce palliative edu-cation into nursing homes is via the link-nurse model, link-nurses could act as a local resource and disseminate information to their colleagues. This could potentially be instrumental to the development of relevant collaborative edu-cational interventions for these workers. The need for inter-professional pal-liative care education, and the recognition of the benefit of inter-professional working on patient care has been endorsed politically, but service users and professionals also promote its advantages. The benefit of inter-professional working is recognised by patient groups as providing the opportunity for bet-ter patient management, which may encourage networking and ultimately improve patient care (Daykin et al., 2002).

An inter-professional approach to education may help students engage in joint consultations and learning, which may facilitate students to appreciate each others' perspectives, and promote an understanding of each other's pro-fessional roles. This synergistic aspect is highlighted by Wakefield et al. (2003), who concluded that encouraging students to interact with each other provides several benefits to the student. This appears to be congruent with the current drive towards inter-professional education and collaborative prac-tice, and validation for this type of educational strategy is particularly appro-priate for palliative care courses, due to the plethora of professionals who work together within this area of practice.

Education in palliative care may require teaching methods that utilise a more reflective and contemplative approach. Pereira et al. (2008) suggest that palliative education should provide other competencies not specific to palliative care, including inter-professional collaboration, holistic care, patient-centred care, self-awareness, humanism, community-based care, and spiritual, religious and cultural sensitivities.

Miyashita et al. (2008) additionally suggest palliative care education should be provided for the general public, as it may dispel misconceptions regarding pain, hydration and end-of life issues, however, the effectiveness of population-based educational interventions is still unclear. Significantly, collaborative working, where local stakeholders, partnerships, minority groups and patient representatives work alongside palliative care educators to promote public education initiatives, may meet this essential and integral dimension for palliative care education.

PRACTICAL APPLICATION OF THE CONCEPT

A one-day communication skills course for non-professionals is held at a regional cancer centre and is offered to any worker within a cancer and palliative care setting. Attendees, primarily, are representative of the myriad of differing workers within cancer and palliative care and, typically, may include healthcare assistants, hospice workers, administrative staff, porters, volunteers, and medical records staff. The course's main content addresses and identifies strategies to enhance communication skills in handling difficult situations. This session is student-led and the agenda for this session is set by the students themselves, who are individually asked to identify an issue or communication difficulty that they have either encountered in practice, or is likely to arise.

To facilitate discussion and identification of effective strategies to handle these identified issues, group discussion and, often, role play is utilised. Student evaluation highlights learning is enhanced by the interactive aspect of the course and appreciation of the differing roles and individual perceptions, which combine to facilitate constructive discussion within the group.

See also: *attributes for palliative caring; communication; environment of care; holism; palliative care and the person with cancer; policy drivers; research in palliative care; value of life*

FURTHER READING

Lloyd-Williams, M. (2003) *Psychosocial Issues in Palliative Care*. Oxford: Oxford University Press.

Faulkner, A. and Maguire, P. (1994) *Talking to Cancer Patients and their Relatives*. Oxford: Oxford Medical Publications.

Foyle, L. and Hostad, J. (2004) *Delivering Cancer and Palliative Care Education*. Oxford: Radcliffe Publishing.

REFERENCES

Banks-Howe, J., Horner, J. and Kelly, C. (2003) 'Educating healthcare support workers in cancer and palliative care', *Cancer Nursing Practice*, 2(10): 35–9.

Blunden, G., Langton, H. and Hek, G. (2001) 'Professional education for the cancer care nurse in England and Wales: a review of the evidence base', *European Journal of Cancer Care*, 10: 179–82.

Daykin, N., Sanidas, M., Barley, V., Evanns, S., McNeill, J., Palmer, N., Rimmer, J., Triiter, J. and Turton, P. (2002) 'Developing consensus and inter-professional working in cancer services; the case for user involvement', *Journal of Inter-professional Care*, 16(4): 405–6.

Foyle, L. and Hostad, J. (2004) *Delivering Cancer and Palliative Care Education*. Oxford: Radcliffe Publishing.

Miyashita, M., Sato, K., Morita, T. and Suzuki, M. (2008) 'Effect of a population based educational intervention focussing on end-of life home care, life prolonging treatment and knowledge about palliative care', *Palliative Care*, 22: 376–82.

National Institute for Clinical Excellence (2004) *Guidance on Cancer Services: Guidelines for Improving Supportive and Palliative Care for Adults with Cancer*. London: NICE.

Pereira, J., Pautex, S., Cantin, B., Gudhat, H., Zaugg, K., Eychmuller, S. and Zulian, G. (2008) 'Palliative care education in Swiss undergraduate medical curricula; a case of too little, too early', *Palliative Medicine*, 22: 730–5.

Richardson, A. (2004) 'Creating a culture of compassion; developing supportive care for people with cancer', *European Journal of Oncology Nursing*, 8: 293–305.

Wakefield, A., Cooke, S. and Boggis, C. (2003) 'Learning together; use of simulated patients with nursing and medical students for breaking bad news', *International Journal of Palliative Nursing*, 9(1): 32–8.

Waldron, M., Hasson, F., Kernohan, W. G., Whittaker, E. and McClaughlin, D. (2008) 'Evaluating education in palliative care with link nurses in nursing homes', *British Journal of Nursing*, 17(1): 1078–83.

33 patient choices and preferences in palliative care

Stephanie Neill and Dorothy Carter

DEFINITION

Much of what is written about patient choices and preferences is from a practitioner's perspective, although what little there is from a patient's perspective is broadly similar. The Liverpool Care Pathway [LCP] (Marie Curie Palliative Care Institute Liverpool) states palliative care is 'To improve the quality of care of the dying in the last hours/days of life'. The *NHS End of*

Life Care Strategy, based upon the LCP, covers the following: being free from pain and comfortable at all times; family, carer and financial needs are dealt with and religious and spiritual values are planned for. Patients are treated with dignity and respect, their wishes are documented and their families are cared for both before and after death.

The findings of a survey from the United States (Steinhauser et al., 2000) about patient preferences asked patients, families, physicians, clergy and hospice volunteers. It showed patients results were broadly similar. It included being able to complete life by saying goodbye, completing unfinished business and having good relationships with doctors and healthcare professionals. Research from Service Users (SUs) receiving palliative care from specialist palliative care social workers (Beresford et al., 2007) showed SUs appreciated their support, found they felt less suicidal, social isolation decreased and felt more in control of their lives.

Because there is so little research from a patient's perspective, we have included four case studies. They are from semi-structured questions with close family members.

CASE STUDY 1

H, aged 83, has lung cancer, which is progressing quite slowly. When she was in hospital recently with pneumonia, her husband, her main carer, died suddenly. She was able to go home with a care package and is doing quite well with support from her family. She is very positive, with full capacity and determined to stay at home as long as possible.

Was she given a diagnosis? Yes. It was very clear, direct and to the point. It was handled very well.

After diagnosis, what choices were given? The right to choose whether or not to have chemotherapy and/or surgery. She chose not to because of her age. There was a multi-disciplinary meeting and after being told all about it, she opted for radiotherapy.

What influenced her choice? The will to live and to keep her dignity.

What were her priorities? To be as pain-free as possible, have family nearby and no resuscitation. The family agreed these choices as well.

Was the treatment fully explained? Yes, but it was difficult to understand. There was not a lot of communication between hospitals.

When did it become palliative? Probably two months after diagnosis.

What were the choices? Home with a care package or residential care. The choice was to be at home with a care package. There was a delay because of procedures but things are now working well. Intermediate or residential care was not on her agenda. H still has full capacity.

Is there anything you would change? Not at the moment. H feels that she is getting good support and the social workers are very good. The hospital ward could maybe have given more information but the OTs and social workers were very informative.

CASE STUDY 2

D was in her late seventies when she started showing the signs of dementia/ Alzheimer's. She managed to stay at home for three years before she was taken ill and hospitalised. She was then referred to an EMI home, where she was happy with the care received as were her family. When she was taken ill with pneumonia, she was sent to the local hospital. After discharge the consultant decided that she was too ill to go to the EMI home and she was sent to a nursing home dealing with mental health issues. The family felt that this was done too quickly, with no discussion about the situation, nor was it properly explained to them. They felt that she had a poor quality of life, they were not consulted and were not given enough information. D's mental and physical condition steadily deteriorated and she was again hospitalised after which she was sent to a general nursing home where she died aged 84.

Do you know what palliative care is? I didn't. I had to work it out for myself. I thought it was just the care of those about to die.

Were you given a diagnosis? Yes – short-term memory loss and effects of ageing. We heard a very good professional give a series of talks and because of this we worked it out for ourselves.

After diagnosis was she given any choices? By then she did not have the capacity to choose for herself and the choices were taken out of our hands as she was taken to a mental health hospital because she was too ill for the EMI home.

Were any choices offered and if so what were they? None. She was sent to a special unit.

What influenced any choices? There weren't any.

What were your priorities? Dignity, a homely atmosphere, where she would feel comfortable, and a caring staff.

When did it become palliative? When she left the home dealing with mental health issues. She stopped eating or perhaps before that.

Did you have any choices about moves that were made? No. The moves were made within days.

Were there any consultations with you? Mostly we were just told. The only consultation was with the older people's consultant but the only option offered was a nursing home.

Were you kept informed at all times? Definitely not. We had to prise it out of them.

When you felt that there were no choices, what did you do? Asked to attend meetings, gained our own information on Alzheimer's. The PCT were not very forthcoming or responsive. The home for mental health issues was helpful, because of my job (I work with people in the community who have mental health issues). The general nursing home was not very good – it was very clinical with very little emotional support. There was a large turnover of staff and personal care was not very good. We don't think a doctor saw her in four months.

If you could change anything, what would it be? She was in four different places in four months, which is too much for an 83-year-old. There should be more information given, less clinical – more emotional care, a more caring attitude shown, more support for families and carers as there were feelings of guilt at not being able to cope. I realised that caring on my own was too much but there was no empathy shown for my feelings. Nursing homes could give better information about their services and choices available. If I had been given a choice, I wouldn't have known which one to choose as there was no information available.

CASE STUDY 3

Jane, a widow aged 88, lived independently in her own home. She had a very close relationship with her only daughter, Pat and her family, who lived close by. Pat worked full-time and her youngest son lived at home.

After two strokes within the last year Jane needed palliative care and was unable to go out alone. She had a great deal of pressure from social workers to go into a home but this meant being some distance away from her family. As Jane's priorities were to retain her independence and be near her family she chose to stay in her own home and have domiciliary care. Care workers would get her up, provide personal care, breakfast and tea, with a night time visit to help her get ready for bed. Jane did all her own cooking and a care worker would do the carrying.

Jane and Pat had quality time in the evening and Pat did heavy cleaning. Her grandsons would pop in during the evenings, which was very important to her. The grandsons would have found it too emotionally gruelling to visit a care home. The care deteriorated and Pat changed agencies twice.

Four years later, Jane was diagnosed with life-threatening diverticulitis and made an informed decision to have surgery. This was the last choice Jane ever made. She was in a surgical ward for four weeks and then moved, without choice, into a discharge ward. No palliative care choices were offered to her. She was not put into a geriatric ward, because there were no beds. The geriatric consultant did not receive the referral.

Her nursing care was extraordinarily poor. Her colostomy bag would detach, and she would sit in its contents for hours. The alarm bell was kept away from her. She was not helped to feed and nurses would be found in their office eating patients' desserts.

Pat demanded her mother had better nursing care and a threat to contact the consultant led to her mother being transferred to the geriatric ward. Here she got very good treatment, but still no choices. At this point Pat stopped eating and faded away. The troublesome surgical ward was closed.

Jane, who had some experience in this field, worked with the directors of nursing on a 13-point plan for palliative care at the hospital. There has been no evidence that this was implemented.

CASE STUDY 4

John was diagnosed with a brain tumour in his mid-fifties, for which surgery and therapies were unsuccessful. He was a big man and as he grew weaker became very difficult to handle. His wife, his main carer, was not in the best of health. Even with a care package, John worried about the strain on his wife, especially if he was ill or fell. He insisted that his wife should have a holiday and went into a residential home for two weeks, where he decided he wanted to stay permanently. He felt he would be looked after and could have quality time with his wife. He went into a nursing home within easy reach of the family home, his wife was able to visit every day and he visited his home once a week.

After a short time they agreed this was working well and that their relationship improved. His wife was able to take him out on excursions or for meals and they had some good times together as she had a lesser caring role. His wife said that she felt lucky because her final memories would be of good quality times, and not the hard work and stress of caring. She had opposed the move to residential care and underwent counselling to help her come to terms with John's decision but eventually she agreed that John's choice was the best for them both. John was pleased that he had been able to make this choice and to have the decision on how to end his days in a dignified way.

The above case studies were conducted, in 2009, by two members of FOCUS (Forum of Carers and Users of Services) who would like to express their gratitude to the interviewees for giving their time and sharing their experiences.

FURTHER READING

Cachia, E. (2007). 'Why Palliative care? Encountering challenging issues', *Malta Medical Journal*, 20(4): 6–10.

Jackson, D., Mula, C. & Coleby, T. (2008) 'Promoting patient choice in end of life care', *Health Service Journal*, 19 September.

National Council for Palliative Care, www.ncpc.org.uk

Preferred Priorities for Care, www.endoflifecare.nhs.uk

Storey, L., Pemberton, C., Howard, A. and O'Donnell, L. (2003) 'Place of death: Hobson's choice or patient choice?' *Cancer Nursing Practice*, 2(4): 33–8.

Sue Ryder Care, Manorlands Hospice (undated). *Involving Service Users*. Sue Ryder Care, Manorlands Hospice.

patient choices and preferences in palliative care

REFERENCES

Beresford, P., Adshead, L., Croft, S. and Rowe, D. (2007) *Palliative Care, Social Work, and Service Users: Making Life Possible*. London: Jessica Kingsley.

FOCUS – Forum of Carers and Users of Services (Identifies, trains and supports service users and carers who are involved in many aspects of Social Work and Health degree courses) Dorothy-focus@O2.co.uk/www.focus-nw.co.uk

Marie Curie Palliative Care Institute Liverpool (MCPCIL) (2008) *What is the LCP? Patient & Carer Overview.* MCPCIL http://www.mcpcil.org.uk/liverpool-care-pathway/pdfs/What%20is%20the%20LCP%20-%20(Patient%20&%20carer%20Overview%20)%20(July%202008)%20(p.pdf) accessed 12 June 2009.

Steinhauser, K.E., Christakis, N.A., Clipp. E.C., McNeilly, M., McIntyre, L. and Tulsky, J. A. (2000) 'Factors considered important at the end of life by patients, family, physicians, and other care providers', *Journal of the American Medical Association*, 284(19): 2476–82.

34 policy drivers

Mzwandile A. Mabhala

DEFINITION

There are several definitions of public policy, but the definition by O'Neill and Pederson (1992) was found to be useful in this context:

> The broad framework of ideas and values within which decisions are taken and action, or inaction, is pursued by governments in relation to some issue or problem.

Central to this definition is the message that policy is more than simply the programmes of a government; it extends beyond the decisions a government chooses to make, and is driven by policy-makers' underpinning political ideologies, principles and values. Thus, public policy is as much a guiding principle as an outcome. This definition further implies that policy can be described as a guiding principle, and not a guarantee, of action.

While the definition refers to social policy, it is resonant with definitions of health policy. The World Health Organisation (WHO) defines health policy as agreement or consensus on the health issues, goals and objectives to be addressed, the priorities among those objectives, and the main directions for achieving them (WHO, 1999).

KEY POINTS

- Policy is as much a guiding principle as an outcome.
- Policy is a guiding principle, not a guarantee, of action.
- Studies have identified social and geographical variations in cancer mortality and incidence, survival and quality of care.
- Subsequent UK policy documents show a change in policy emphasis from access to service to quality and choice.

DISCUSSION

Public health challenges alter as populations change and causes of morbidity and mortality shift. Over the past century in developed countries, longevity has improved, largely because of public health improvements. The causes of death have changed, altering the nature of death: more people are dying from serious chronic diseases rather than acute illnesses. The consequences of this shifting landscape have been a shift in health policy and a redefinition of public health in line with the changing demographic context and disease and health trends.

HM Treasury (2004: 26) presents a modern definition (one coined by Sir Donald Acheson) of public health informing policy in the UK: 'The science and art of preventing disease, prolonging life, and promoting health through the organised efforts of society.' This definition is widely used because it reflects the essential elements of modern public health – a population perspective, an emphasis on collective responsibility for health and on prevention, and the key role of the state linked to concern for the underlying socio-economic determinants of health (HM Treasury, 2004). It encapsulates a belief in social justice as the foundation for public health practice. It also embraces the view that public health is a population issue, as opposed to an individual matter, and that conceptions of equity and fairness held by a society at any given time are captured by a portrait of the distribution of health and disease across the various groups that comprise it. Notions of fairness and equitable access to health provision have been core principles of UK health policy, signified by a number of policy initiatives to improve access to primary care services and tackle health inequalities.

Alongside UK government commitments to the development of a primary care-led NHS (Department of Health, 2004a), the provision of cancer and palliative care services and programmes for terminally ill patients has become an important public health issue in recent decades (Department of Health, 2004a, 2007). However, despite the increasing recognition of palliative care and health inequalities as major public health challenges, a plethora of evidence shows remarkable geographic variation in the availability and provision of palliative care services. For example, several studies have consistently indicated that UK cancer patients are less likely to receive palliative care if they have low socio-economic status (SES) (Gatrell et al., 2003; Currin et al.,

2009). These variations have been attributed to UK specialist palliative care frequently being provided by the voluntary sector in conjunction with the National Health Service. These services often serve a small, often privileged, proportion of society comprising patients dying of malignancies, and living in deprived geographical areas. Despite policy recognition of primary care professionals as providers of palliative care, the processes, resources and skills to provide effective palliative care are often lacking (Dale et al., 2009). This view was acknowledged when a government review of NHS spending stated that government's commitment to primary care has not been matched by increases in resources, improvements in health across the socio-economic spectrum and a policy focus on the wider economic determinants of health (HM Treasury, 2004).

Successive policy documents, such as *Choosing Health* (Department of Health, 2004b), responded to these imbalances by reinforcing the message of choice, reflecting a new recognition that no amount of legislation, regulation or structural adjustment can compete with the ability of people to choose how they live their lives. Notions of choice and personalised care seem to offer promising prospects for families and palliative care patients. The evidence suggests that for many people, home is more than a physical space; it represents familiarity, the presence of loved ones, and the possibility of enjoying 'normal' life – reasons why well over half of the people with progressive illness want to die at home (Gomes and Higginson, 2006). Reality suggests otherwise; evidence reported in the WHO (2004) analysis of palliative care showed that, even though their choice is to die at home, most people in the UK, the US, Germany, Switzerland, and France die in hospitals. In the UK, the proportion of home deaths for patients with cancer is falling, from 27% in 1994 to 22% in 2003.

Furthermore, several studies examined predictors of place of death among those with cancer; these studies show compelling evidence that up to 70% of people with cancer prefer to die at home (Grande et al., 1998). The results from these studies consistently show correlation between SES and quality of palliative care provision; in more deprived areas, cancer patients are more likely to die in hospital or hospice, and less likely to die at home (Gatrell et al., 2003; Gomes and Higginson, 2006). At the individual level, probability of death at home decreases among those in deprived areas, whereas probability of death in hospital increases.

Promoting health, prevention of disease, prolonging life and tackling inequalities in health are key public health strategies, but ethically we should not overlook the multitude of people who are already suffering while we plan for the future. Clearly there are great inequalities in provision of palliative care services. It would appear that the need for palliative care is a public health issue, which public health practitioners and health policy makers may not be prioritizing. This is one of several public health issues that deserve priority; and is one that is currently being neglected in public health discussions.

PRACTICAL APPLICATION OF THE CONCEPT

Our condolences go to Mrs Zuma's and Mrs Van Wyk's families and to the Wyngaart Accounting Firm, and the Baptist Church for the loss of two of its valuable members within one year.

Mrs Zuma was a cleaner in the Wyngaart Accounting Firm and Baptist Church leader; Mrs Van Wyk was a chief accountant and member of the Baptist Church. Both were diagnosed with cervical cancer. In her last days of her battle with cancer Mrs Van Wyk requested to die in her home; this request was granted and she received all her palliative care at home among close friends and family.

Mrs Zuma, as a church leader, paid regular visits for spiritual support. She was impressed with this model of care. At the advanced stage of her condition she also requested health and social services to arrange her care to be delivered in her home. This request was granted, but they admitted her to hospice care while the home package was being set up. Unfortunately she later died in the hospice while still waiting for her home package to be installed.

See also: environment of care; palliative care and the person with cancer

REFERENCES

Currin, L.G., Jack, R.H., Linklater, K.M., Mak, V., Moller, H. and Davies, E.A. (2009) 'Inequalities in the incidence of cervical cancer in South East England 2001–2005: an investigation of population risk factors', *BMC Public Health*, 9(62): 1–10.

Dale, J., Petrova, M., Munday, D., Koistinen-Harris, J., Lall, R. and Thomas, K. (2009) 'A national facilitation project to improve primary palliative care: impact of the Gold Standards Framework on process and self-ratings of quality', *Quality & Safety in Health Care*, 18(34): 174–80.

Department of Health (2004a) *The NHS Cancer Plan and the New NHS: Providing a Patient-centred Service*. London: Department of Health.

Department of Health (2004b) *Choosing Health: Making Healthier Choices Easier*. London: Department of Health.

Department of Health (2007) *Cancer Reform Strategy*. London: Department of Health.

Gatrell, A.C., Harman, J.C., Francis, B.J., Thomas, C., Morris, S.M. and McIllmurray, T. (2003) 'Place of death: analysis of cancer deaths in part of North West England', *Journal of Public Health Medicine*, 25(1): 53–8.

Gomes, B. and Higginson, I.J. (2006) 'Factors influencing death at home in terminally ill patients with cancer: systematic review', *British Medical Journal*, 332(7540): 515–8).

Grande, G.E., Addington-Hall, J. and Todd, C.J. (1998) 'Place of death and access to home care services: are certain patient groups at a disadvantage?', *Social Science & Medicine*, 47(5): 565–79.

HM Treasury (2004) *Securing Good Health for the Whole Population*. London: Treasury Office.

O'Neill, M. & Pederson, A. (1992) 'Building a methods bridge between policy analysis and healthy public policy', *Canadian Journal of Public Health*, 83(supplement 1): 25–30.

World Health Organisation (1999) *Health 21: The Health for All Policy Frameworks for the WHO European Region*. Copenhagen: World Health Organisation regional office for Europe, pp. 2–3.

World Health Organisation (2004) *Better Palliative Care for Older People*. Available at: www. euro.who.int/InformationSources/Publications/Catalogue/20050118_2, accessed 16 June 2009.

35 quality assurance and palliative care

Jill McCarthy

DEFINITION

Quality assurance in health care is concerned with promoting the best care available and delivering this in a timely and cost effective manner. This is achieved through an ongoing cycle of monitoring, evaluating and improving health care delivery by such mechanisms as audit of services, risk assessments, peer reviews and research studies. Quality assurance should be an essential component of all health care delivery and palliative care is no exception to this. However, the word quality is in itself nebulous, for example, this may mean compassionate and timely care to a patient, effective clinical performance to a health care professional and cost effective care delivery to a care purchaser (Ingleton and Faulkner, 1995). This confusion is further compounded in palliative care whereby traditional indicators of quality, such as death or recovery rates, are not appropriate and the ultimate goal may not be an improvement in the overall condition of the patient but, in some cases, the achievement of a good death. There is also, with palliative care, the sensitive matter of assessing patient satisfaction with services, when patients may be terminally ill or dying, and seeking answers from carers or recently bereaved relatives may provide conflicting views from those of the patient, giving results that are skewed.

KEY POINTS

- Quality assurance is an essential component of palliative care.
- It is concerned with promoting the best care in a timely and cost effective way.

- The word *quality* is indistinct.
- Quality in palliative care may refer to a good death.
- Patient satisfaction with palliative care services may be difficult to ascertain.

DISCUSSION

Palliative care in the United Kingdom is a comparatively new concept, having emerged in the 1960s as a response to the lack of adequate physical and psychological treatment of terminally ill people (Bruera, 1996). In order to increase mainstream recognition and funding of palliative care service to provide further access for patients and families and further education for health care professionals, it is important that these services demonstrate crucial, cost effective care. Quality assurance provides the mechanisms to validate palliative care delivery. As traditional quality indicators are not always appropriate in palliative care, it is important to establish alternative approaches to measuring the quality of care services and interventions. McWhinney et al. (1994: 1340) note how difficulties arise in evaluating services because of 'attrition due to early death, opposition to randomisation by patients and referral sources, ethical problems raised by randomisation of dying patients, the appropriate timing of comparison points, and difficulties of collecting data from sick or exhausted patients and care givers'. However, evaluation of services undertaken by qualitative studies, surveys and audits has proved to be more effective, although the challenge of collecting data from sick and dying patients remains unchanged.

In recent years the Government has been involved in a series of initiatives in relation to palliative care services, all of which have provided quality assurance mechanisms or guidance from which quality can be assessed. These can be seen as a direct result of the The NHS Cancer Plan (Department of Health, 2000) that demonstrated how community cancer services were often not as good as they could be, for example, many patients with advanced cancer stated that they would prefer to die at home, but in reality only approximately 25% of these did so. In addition, the *Cancer Patient Survey* (Department of Health, 2002a) that recorded the experiences of patients who had received hospital care for cancer as an in-patient or day case in 1999/2000 revealed marked differences in care across diagnoses and across trusts, indicating the need for robust quality assurance mechanisms to be put in place.

In 2007, the Government produced the *Gold Standards Framework for Palliative Care* (National Health Service, 2007) that is designed to improve the palliative care received by patients nearing the end of their lives. It is intended to be used primarily by people who are being cared for in the community by primary health care teams. In addition to the Gold Standards Framework, the Department of Health has launched the *End of Life Care Strategy* (Department of Health, 2008) as a benchmark to help improve the quality of care for terminally ill people across the care sectors. This document recommends that the needs of terminally ill patients are assessed in order to provide pertinent palliative treatment and care, as well as support for relatives, carers and friends. Care home managers are required to have policies and procedures in place for care of their terminally ill or dying residents which meet the *National Minimum Standards* (Department of Health, 2002b) relating to palliative care. In addition, it is recommended that doctors are annually assessed and required to revalidate their licence under General Medical Council standards based on the *Good Medical Practice* framework (General Medical Council, 2006), which includes issues related to palliative care and dying.

In an effort to provide research-based palliative care delivery, many trusts are also utilising an Integrated Care Pathway for the Care of the Dying, which is an evidence-based document that acts as a framework to guide care professionals. It is designed to prompt and lead appropriate actions such as symptom management, psychosocial issues and communication with patients and their families, alongside the promotion of multi-disciplinary discussions. Care pathways for the care of the dying person are now part of the Gold Standards Framework in the community, and implementation is recommended in the National Institute for Clinical Excellence guidance on *Improving Supportive and Palliative Care for Adults with Cancer* (NICE, 2004) for both acute and community settings. In addition, professional bodies have produced specific guidance for their clinicians working in palliative care, for example, the Royal College of Nursing (2002) and the General Medical Council (2006). All of these initiatives provide benchmarks from which quality can be monitored, evaluated and, when necessary, improved.

Ferris (2004: 750) poses the question 'Do standards and guidelines in palliative care matter?' going on to state that there is a 'mounting frenzy' to produce these. Standards and guidelines are produced in an attempt to provide consistency across the service spectrum, ensuring quality no matter where the palliative care is delivered. However, 'there needs to be a clear perspective and application strategy so that we don't end up with a biblical Tower of Babel instead of a clear way forward that enhances the field' (Ferris, 2004: 750). Presently it can be seen that there are a plethora of quality assurance initiatives in the palliative care arena but, as stated previously, these can sometimes prove difficult to evaluate. Bruera (1996: 157) recommends that we not only ask the question 'Are we doing things well?' in palliative care, but also the question 'Are we doing things right?'

Quality assurance in palliative care is of the utmost importance, and must underpin all care delivery systems. The quality of care provided is dependent upon an understanding of the underlying philosophy that is guiding this care delivery by all concerned. Implementation of quality palliative care commences with careful strategic planning followed by the systematic development of guidelines, outcome measures, indicators, standards and a performance improvement process. Quality assurance in palliative care provides patients with the best evidence-based treatments and ensures that they and their families will be regarded as individuals who are treated with dignity and respect and involved in all decision-making surrounding their treatment and care.

PRACTICAL APPLICATION OF THE CONCEPT

Susan is a 56-year-old married woman who was previously diagnosed with breast cancer and underwent a mastectomy operation and further treatment. However, she has not been feeling well during the last month and on referral to her oncology consultant, she and her husband are given the devastating news that the cancer has spread and the prognosis is poor.

Susan is referred to the Macmillan services and a nurse visits Susan at her home. The nurse delicately discusses Susan's prognosis with her and Susan finds that it is a huge relief to be able to talk openly about the fact that she is going to die. Susan does not want to go into a hospital or hospice and the nurse reassures her that she can remain in her own home to die, and that her relatives will be well supported by the primary health care team and any pain will be well controlled.

As her condition deteriorates, the district nurses and general practitioner become more involved with Susan's care. During the last few days of her life, she is put onto an Integrated Care Pathway for the Care of the Dying and she dies peacefully at home surrounded by her family, in accordance with her last wishes.

See also: *agencies; finance issues and the organisation of palliative care; good death; patient choice and preferences in palliative care; research in palliative care*

FURTHER READING

LaPorte Matzo, M. and Witt Sherman, D. (eds) (2005) *Palliative Care Nursing: Quality Care to the End of Life*, 2nd edn. New York: Springer Publishing Co.

Lynn, J., Chaudhry, E., Simon, L.N., Wilkinson A.M. and Schuster, J.N. (2007) *The Common Sense Guide to Improving Palliative Care*. Oxford: Oxford University Press.

Payne, S., Seymour, J. and Ingleton, C. (eds) (2008) *Palliative Care Nursing. Principles and Evidence for Practice*, 2nd edn. Maidenhead: Open University Press.

REFERENCES

Bruera, E. (1996) 'Quality assurance in palliative care – a growing "must"' Editorial, *Support Care Cancer*, 4: 157.

Department of Health (2000) *The NHS Cancer Plan: A Plan for Investment, A Plan for Reform*. London: Department of Health.

Department of Health (2002a) *Cancer Patient Survey. NHS Cancer Plan: A Baseline Survey*. London: Department of Health.

Department of Health (2002b) *Independent Health Care: National Minimum Standards Regulations*. London: Department of Health.

quality assurance

165

Department of Health (2008) *End of Life Care Strategy: Promoting High Quality Care for All Adults at the End of Life*. London: Department of Health.

Ferris, F.D. (2004) 'Standards and guidelines: Do they matter?', *Journal of Palliative Care*, 7(6): 750–2.

General Medical Council (2006) *Good Medical Practice*. London: GMC.

Ingleton, C. and Faulkner, A. (1995) 'Quality assurance in cancer care: some of the problems', *European Journal of Cancer Care*, 4: 38–44.

McWhinney, I.R., Bass, M.J. and Donner, A. (1994) 'Evaluation of a palliative care service: problems and pitfalls', *British Medical Journal*, 19(309): 1340–2.

National Health Service (2007) '*The Gold Standards Framework: A Programme for Community Palliative Care*, available at: www.goldstandardsframework.nhs.uk/, accessed 18 May 2009.

National Institute for Clinical Excellence (2004) *Guidance on Cancer Services: Improving Supportive and Palliative Care for Adults with Cancer*. London: NICE.

Royal College of Nursing (2002) *Competencies in Nursing: A Framework for Nurses Working in Specialist Palliative Care. Competencies Project*. London: RCN.

36 reactions of patients and carers

key concepts in palliative care

166

Sue Phillips

DEFINITION

This concept explores the way in which individuals react to news of terminal illness. Reactions: 'A response to some treatment, situation or stimulus'. Responses differ depending on many things – culture, personality, emotional maturity, coping strategies, age, religion, and existence of significant loving others (Kang et al., 2006).

KEY POINTS

- People react in very different ways to terminal illness.
- Typical reactions include tearfulness, guilt, anger, denial, stoic acceptance, bargaining and depression.
- Health professionals need to be aware of the range of reactions, and to respond sensitively.

DISCUSSION

Individuals' reactions to terminal illness will be very different, although common themes will emerge. News such as this will, of course, affect both patients and carers, and again, will differ, depending on personality and circumstances. Psychological and physical responses to terminal illness, such as depression, fear and anxiety, differ according to emotional maturity, coping strategies, cultural environment, religion, age, stage of illness, and existence of loving family and friends (National Comprehensive Cancer Network, 2008). Kübler-Ross (1970) described five reactions to impending loss – denial, anger, bargaining, depression and acceptance. Kübler-Ross's stages should not be interpreted too literally, as people may move between the stages in an unpredictable way, and often these stages provide a defence to help individuals cope at a time of great personal stress. There are other responses and reactions to terminal illness, and some of these will be explored in more depth.

Depression and anxiety

A depressed mood can be characterised as feelings of worthlessness or excessive guilt, diminished interest or pleasure in usual activities, suicidal thoughts, and a preoccupation with death (Kang et al., 2006) Depression can be related to anticipatory grief of impending loss of life, increased physical impairment, pain, and hopelessness. This is related to fear and anxiety. Anxiety is an emotion experienced by most patients in different stages of their terminal illness (Lugton, 2002). One of the most prevalent feelings when someone is diagnosed with a life-threatening condition is fear (Costello, 2004). This fear includes anxiety about the type of death, pain and suffering, and a series of 'what if?' questions. This fear may also include fear of what may happen to loved ones, children, for example, when they are no longer there to care for them. The causes of depression are therefore multi-faceted, and health professionals need to bear this in mind when considering appropriate treatment for a patient who is depressed.

Guilt or blame

Patients or carers may feel guilty that the illness is a punishment for past sins or, alternatively, blame, a belief that the current situation is the fault of others (Faulkner, 1998). Patients may feel guilty about the demands that they have to make on their care-giver, or that they've become a burden to their families. Relatives may feel that they cannot express any negative feelings about people because they are dying, and may feel guilty for even thinking them. This may mean that relationships may become distorted at a time when they are of paramount importance. Self-awareness and sensitive communication skills are needed by healthcare professionals to try to understand and work through some of these reactions with patients and their carers.

Denial

Denial may be a valid coping mechanism for those who are unable or not yet ready to adapt to the reality of a terminal illness (Faulkner, 1998). Denial is generally considered to be unconscious and unapparent to the person using it as a method of coping, although occasionally the patient may *choose* to deny their impending death (Zimmerman, 2004). In the short term, denial can be an adaptive coping strategy; it can protect someone from the full implications of what has happened. In other words, it can be a gradual means of coming to terms with the situation (Kübler-Ross, 1970). In the longer term, however, denial can cause problems; for example, dying patients may refuse treatment which may help them, such as pain relief. Also, if relatives deny that patients are dying, it can lead to friction with staff, who have their patients' best interests at heart. Health professionals working in palliative care are in a unique position to manage and influence the dying process, including encouraging the psychological adaptation to the label of 'dying.'

Anger

Seriously ill people and their relatives may show a lot of anger or aggression (Kübler-Ross, 1970). Often this disguises underlying fears or anxieties. Patients may express anger against their illness, for example, that a cancer has metastasised (Chunlestskul et al., 2008), or anger at God for allowing them to become ill, or not being healed. If a person's anger is directed against relatives or health professionals, it may discourage them from trying to help, thus leaving the patient lonely and isolated. Sometimes anger shows itself in constant complaints about treatment and care. There may be good reason for the anger, for example, delay in making a diagnosis. Health professionals need to explore aspects of the reality that is causing the anger and expectations about care and treatment discussed.

Stoicism

Occasionally, a patient's or carer's reaction seems to be inappropriately stoical. This may be the case in the later stages of a terminal illness, when grief and distress have been worked through at an earlier stage, and the patient has come to accept the likely outcome of their illness. It may also be evident in individuals with a religious faith, in that they may see the illness as something which is sent to test them (McGrath, 2003). Webb and Koch (1997: 519) describe the principal reaction of women diagnosed with breast cancer as a 'calm acceptance of something about which they could do nothing and about which it was, therefore, not worth getting upset'. The researchers found this surprising, but could identify no cultural or other specific reason for this response. The implications for health professionals are that they should not interpret this non-reaction as a lack of patient concern or worry. In some cases, some individuals go on to exhibit distress by other means, for example, an increased reporting of physical symptoms, additional non-verbal communication of pain (Travaline et al., 2005).

PRACTICAL APPLICATION OF THE CONCEPT.

My family has never been one for displaying our emotions openly. Sometimes this is hard for others to understand, and my mother would sometimes feel the need to explain that she had her own way of 'dealing with things'. My sister had been treated, we hoped successfully, for breast cancer. However, she was admitted to hospital suddenly in the night about 18 months following her initial diagnosis, when she had a fit. I knew that this was likely to mean bad news, that the cancer had spread. She was discharged from hospital, and sent a follow-up outpatient appointment. Her husband refused to go with her; I wasn't sure whether he was in denial or genuinely did not appreciate the seriousness of her condition. I suspect the former. So I went to the appointment with my sister. We were told that she had secondaries in her brain, and that there was very limited treatment available. Neither of us cried, and in fact accepted the information in a very stoic way. When we left the consulting room, I was called back on my own to see the doctors. They had thought from our reaction that we had not understood the seriousness of my sister's condition, and were keen to emphasise that she had four metastases and her condition was terminal.

When I drove my sister home, we made some tea. Her only comment was that she would have liked to see her four children grow up. Neither of us cried.

Reflecting back, my main reaction was an excessive tiredness, extreme weariness, moments of grief and anger, but overall, a stoic acceptance, coupled with anxiousness for her husband and family.

See also: communication; loss, grief and bereavement;

FURTHER READING

Brown, C. (2009) 'Cancergiggles', in S. Earle, C. Bartholomew and C. Komaromy (eds) *Making Sense of Death, Dying and Bereavement: An Anthology.* London: Sage.

Mitchell, G., Murray, J., and Hynson, J. (2008) 'Understanding the whole person: life-limiting illness across the life cycle', in G. Mitchell (ed.) *Palliative Care: A Patient Centered Approach.* Oxford: Radcliffe.

REFERENCES

Chunlestskul, K., Carlson, L.E., Koopmans, J.P. and Angen., M.J. (2008) 'Lived experiences of Canadian women with metastatic breast cancer in preparation for their death: a qualitative study', *Journal of Palliative Care,* 24(1): 5–17.

Costello, J., (2004) *Nursing the Dying Patient.* Basingstoke: Palgrave-Macmillan.

reactions of patients and carers

169

Faulkner, A. (1998) 'Communication with patients, families and other professionals', *British Medical Journal*, 316: 130–2.

Kang, K.A., Miller, J.R. and Lee W. H. (2006) 'Psychological responses to terminal illness and eventual death in Koreans with cancer', *Research and Theory for Nursing Practice: An International Journal*, 20(1): 29–47.

Kübler-Ross E. (1970) *On Death and Dying.* London: Tavistock.

Lugton J. (2002) *Communicating with Dying People and their Relatives.* Oxford: Radcliffe.

McGrath, P. (2003) 'Religiosity and the challenge of terminal illness', *Death Studies*, 27: 881–99.

National Comprehensive Cancer Network (2008) *NCCN Practice Guidelines for the Management of Psychosocial Distress.* Available at: www.nccn.org/professionals/physician_gls/PDF/distress.pdf, accessed 3 March 2009.

Travaline, J.M., Ruchinskas R. and D'Alonzo G.E. (2005) 'Patient–physician communication: why and how', *Journal of the American Osteopathic Association*, 105(1): 13–18.

Webb, C. and Koch, T. (1997) 'Women's experiences of non-invasive breast cancer: literature review and study report', *Journal of Advanced Nursing*, 25: 514–25.

Zimmerman, C. (2004) 'Denial of impending death: a discourse analysis of the palliative care literature', *Social Science & Medicine*, 59: 1769–80.

37 rehabilitation in palliative care

Claire Jones and Adrian Bunnell

DEFINITION

You matter because you are you and you matter until the last moment of your life. We will do all we can not only to help you to die peacefully but also to live until you die. (Saunders, 1976: 1003)

Rehabilitation can be defined as restoring to former position, putting back in good condition or helping to adjust to normal conditions. This implies restoration to previous ability, which, in the case of patients with palliative care needs, is not always possible. There is little consensus on the definition of rehabilitation. Young et al. (1999) suggest the term rehabilitation is used in a restricted sense, referring to a discreet, time-limited, period of therapy, aimed at restoring power or function. The objective of the rehabilitative approach is to promote a partnership between the healthcare professional and the patient. While rehabilitation and palliative care may appear to be at opposite ends of the spectrum, the World Health Organisation's definition of palliative care (World Health Organisation, 1990) advocates offering a support system to help patients to live actively until death. The whole concept of rehabilitation in palliative care has gained support following the report by the Department of Health Advisory Group on Rehabilitation (Department of Health, 1997). Certainly there appears to be a contradiction between the conventional principles of rehabilitation and the concept of palliative care. However, with appropriate intervention, mobility levels can be maintained and available functional ability utilised, enabling a patient to remain independent for as long as the disease process allows.

KEY POINTS

Rehabilitation in palliative care needs:

- to be patient-led rehabilitation;
- goals set by patient, their carers and the therapist;
- realistic, achievable, short-term goals;
- goals constantly revisited as condition progresses;
- emphasis on enabling rather than restoration of function;
- to maintain hope without giving false expectations.

DISCUSSION

The NICE guidance on supportive and palliative care (NICE, 2004), recommends that rehabilitation be available to all patients with palliative care needs no matter what the stage of their disease. The National Service Frameworks for Long Term Conditions (Department of Health, 2005) and for Older People (Department of Health, 2001), and the NICE Guidelines for Supportive and Palliative Care (NICE, 2004) all emphasise the importance of rehabilitation and enabling patients to live with their disease.

Rehabilitation does not necessarily imply the restoration of function to a premorbid level but does involve maintaining a degree of control and self-esteem. Patient involvement in their own rehabilitation is critical, as it is directly associated with maintenance of dignity, autonomy and compliance with treatment programmes. Patients should be encouraged to recognise their own needs thereby achieving a degree of ownership of jointly agreed goals. This is as relevant in a palliative care setting as in any other speciality (Corner, 2002).

An awareness of a patient's diagnosis and prognosis is important when planning treatment. If goal setting is to be realistic, holistic and achievable, it must be guided by the presenting functional deficits and symptoms which often include overwhelming fatigue. In order to accommodate such problems, the assessment process may require modification over a longer period. Symptom control, together with psychological and pastoral care, is seen as imperative for truly holistic palliative care, with rehabilitation often being regarded as a secondary issue. The value of symptom control can be limited if patients' functional abilities are not addressed, for example, when they are bedbound or bored. Rehabilitation has been described as making the patient into a person again who is useful, creative and feels valued. Hope underpins the whole rehabilitation process of enabling patients to gain control over their own situation. Patients can be over-ambitious, believing the harder they work, the fitter they become, creating false hope. Conversely, some can be in despair not wanting to co-operate, in effect having given up. All patients have to balance their ability with their disability, a situation which varies on a daily basis (Fulton and Else, 1998).

Mackey (2000) suggests enabling a patient to retain some independence might enhance quality of life and assist in maintaining self-identity. There is a delicate balance between providing 'total care' for patients with palliative care needs and promoting independence, as it is possible to provide too much care thus stripping them of their decision-making, autonomy and impairing rehabilitation potential. Rehabilitation in palliative care has been described as 'rehabilitation in reverse' (Pizzi and Briggs, 2006: 125). It may be that an initial goal for a patient is to walk to the bathroom independently. As the patient's condition deteriorates, this goal may change to walking to the bathroom with a walking aid and a carer, and then to being able to transfer safely onto a commode at the side of the bed. While progress appears to be in reverse and the general trend is downwards, the patient is still given positive rehabilitation goals to achieve. The aims are to ensure safety and maintain quality of life for as long as the condition allows.

Cummings (1998) acknowledges that the complexity of issues faced by patients and their families, who are confronted with a palliative diagnosis, exceeds the skills of any single profession. Support can be offered by the entire rehabilitation team to arrive at a situation of realistic achievement. Multi-professional team working diminishes such problems where issues, including rehabilitation needs, are commonly addressed. Listening and providing emotional support are key elements in palliative care rehabilitation and may be seen as outside of the normal scope of practice of the traditional therapy team. There has to be an element of transferring and sharing of skills between professionals to ensure the needs of the patient are met. This holistic approach ensures whole team communication. Where professionals are mindful of each other's goals, inter-professional trust is encouraged, thus facilitating a willingness to share skills among team members allowing collaborative practice. Such an example is where nursing staff continue a mobility and exercise programme between therapy visits.

Traditional rehabilitation services are commonly evaluated by means of outcome measures which can provide measurable, quantifiable values on the success of services. In palliative care this is often difficult as the overall trend of patients' progress is inevitably downwards. By ensuring that goals are small and achievable, it is often possible to measure a positive outcome of therapeutic intervention.

Rehabilitation is as important in the field of palliative care as it is in any other branch of medicine. People with life-limiting illnesses should be afforded the same rehabilitation opportunities as any other patient group. They must be enabled to maximise their remaining functional abilities in order that they are able to work towards any unfulfilled goals.

PRACTICAL APPLICATION OF THE CONCEPT

Peter was a 32-year-old father of two young children, aged 5 and 9. Peter was a self-employed window cleaner and his wife, Julie, was a shop assistant. Julie noticed that Peter had developed an unusually high stepping gait and was tending to trip when walking. When his speech became slightly slurred, she persuaded him to see his GP. Motor neurone disease was diagnosed at the regional neurological centre with a subsequent referral to the community palliative therapy team. He was assessed by the multi-professional team at various stages throughout his illness and a number of rapidly changing goals and actions were identified. Table 37.1 highlights some of these goals over the ensuing months.

Table 37.1 Patient goal sheet

Date	Problem	Goal	Action
22/01/08	Decreased muscle power all 4 limbs.	Maintain function for as long as disease allows.	General exercise programme adapted cutlery/toothbrush/ pen to compensate for reduced grip.
22/01/08	Anticipates not being able to work. Worried about loss of role.	Obtain financial advice. Support patient as he comes to terms with his losses.	Refer to Motor Neurone Disease Association for support for the whole family. Link in to hospice social worker for benefits advice.
15/02/08	Patient at risk of tripping due to weak dorsiflexors and drop foot.	Minimise the risk of injury through falls.	Dorsiflexion exercises and stretches with theraband. Supply with walking stick to aid balance. Progress to crutches/walking frame as condition progresses. Refer to orthotist for drop foot orthoses. Supply with bath lift.
15/02/08	Patient developing slurred speech.	Ensure patient is given appropriate advice on managing bulbar problems.	Refer to speech therapist.

(Continued)

Table 37.1   (Continued)

Date	Problem	Goal	Action
25/05/08	Further deterioration of muscle power in all four limbs. Struggling with mobility, transfers and personal activities of daily living.	Enable patient to cope with activities of daily living for as long as possible. Maintain/improve quality of life.	Refer for electric wheelchair, "closomat" toilet, "neater-eater", ramp. Advise on optimal positioning to facilitate use of remaining functional movement. Teach family/carers safe transfers and use of hoist. Adapt bed and teach alternative transfer techniques.
13/06/08	Increasing bulbar symptoms. Patient at risk of aspiration pneumonia.	Reduce the risk of aspiration.	Re-refer to speech therapist for discussions around swallowing and possibility of peg feed. Advise on positioning to reduce risk of aspiration. Refer to GP for Hyoscine patches to dry secretions. Teach forced expiratory technique and supported coughing. Supply with suction machine and teach family/carers how to use.
19/08/08	Unable to change own sitting/lying position. At risk of pressure sores.	Reduce the risk of complications associated with prolonged bed rest.	Arrange supply of electric profiling bed and pressure relieving mattress.

Table 37.1 illustrates the complexity of problems encountered by this patient, his family and the therapy team. Owing to rapid deterioration it is often necessary to anticipate problems before they arise to prevent crisis situations developing. It is important to maintain a balance between timely intervention and the destruction of hope. Peter and Julie were guided to help them to foresee possible future problems and allow adaptations and equipment to be ordered in good time to maintain independence without increasing their fear for the future. Peter was enabled to optimise his quality of life and ultimately, to die in his preferred place of care, his own home, with his family around him.

See also: *holism; technology*

FURTHER READING

Long, A.F., Kneafsey, R., Ryan, J. and Berry, J. (2002) 'The role of the nurse within the multi-professional rehabilitation team', *Journal of Advanced Nursing*, 37(1): 70–8.
National Council for Palliative Care (2006) *Fulfilling Lives: Rehabilitation in Palliative Care. A Briefing Update*. London: NCPC.

Oldervoll, L.M., Loge, J.H., Paltiel, H., Asp, M.B., Vidvei, U., Hjermstad, M.J. & Kaasa, S. (2005) 'Are palliative cancer patients willing and able to participate in a physical exercise programme?', *Palliative and Supportive Care*, 3(4): 281–87.

Quinn, H., Allan, H. and Bryan, K. (2004) 'An evaluation of a dependency assessment: experiences of staff, patients and carers in a UK hospice', *International Journal of Palliative Nursing*, 10(12): 592–9.

REFERENCES

Corner, J. (2002) 'Self management in palliative care', *International Journal of Palliative Nursing*, 8(11): 516.

Cummings, I. (1998) 'The interdisciplinary team', in D. Doyle, G. Hanks and N. MacDonald (eds), *Oxford Textbook of Palliative Medicine*, 2nd edn. Oxford: Oxford University Press, pp. 19–30.

Department of Health (1997) *Rehabilitation – a Guide* (NHS Executive). London: Department of Health.

Department of Health (2001) *National Service Framework for Older People*. London: Department of Health.

Department of Health (2005) *National Service Framework for Long Term Conditions*. London: Department of Health.

Fulton, C.L. and Else, R. (1998) 'Physiotherapy', in D. Doyle, G. Hanks, and N. MacDonald (eds), *Oxford Textbook of Palliative Medicine*, 2nd edn. Oxford: Oxford University Press, pp. 819–28.

Mackey, K. (2000) 'Experiences of older women with cancer receiving hospice care: significance for physical therapy', *Physical Therapy*, 80(5): 459–68.

NICE (2004) *Supportive and Palliative Care Guidelines*. London: National Institute for Clinical Excellence.

Pizzi, M.A. and Briggs, R. (2006) 'Occupational and physical therapy in a hospice: the facilitation of meaning, quality of life and well-being', *Topics in Geriatric Rehabilitation*, 20(2): 120–30.

Saunders, C., (1976) 'Care of the dying-1: the problem of euthanasia', *Nursing Times*, 72: 1003–5.

World Health Organisation (WHO) (1990) *Cancer, Pain Relief and Palliative Care*. Technical report series 804. Geneva: World Health Organisation.

Young, J., Brown, A., Forster, A. and Clare, J. (1999) 'An overview of rehabilitation for older people', *Reviews in Gerontology*, 9: 181–96.

rehabilitation in palliative care

38 research in palliative care

Catherine Black

DEFINITION

Palliative care is a vital aspect of all areas of health care and, as such, requires a firm base of evidence to support the clinical decisions made and interventions offered. Research can be seen as a systematic way of examining the information available to answer a particular question, or gather more information in order to describe a phenomenon more accurately. It may take many forms, for example, randomised controlled trials, cohort studies, case studies, but to be worthwhile the methodology must be appropriate for the subject being studied and the data collection and analysis should be rigorous.

Dean and McClement (2002) identify eight broad areas worthy of research within the palliative care field. These are: symptoms; ethics; clinical decision-making; communications; family and family care giving issues; inter-disciplinary team issues; health systems and services and existential and spiritual concerns. Their list extends the areas for research from those directly concerning the patient, to include wider sociological and service delivery issues. More recently, Perkins et al. (2008) asked terminally ill hospice patients their priorities for research. The three most important issues identified were: finding ways to ensure that patients knew who to contact in emergencies; discovering better ways to manage pain; discovering better ways to help doctors to hear and understand their patients. These findings show that patients' priorities may differ from those of the professionals.

This difficulty of focus within the research can be compounded by the problem of defining the patient population to be studied (Grande and Ingleton, 2008). Palliative care is a wide ranging concept that includes many long term conditions from the point of diagnosis such as Chronic Obstructive Pulmonary Disease (COPD), multiple sclerosis, motor neurone disease and cancer. This non-specific concept does not help the palliative care researcher to identify appropriate inclusion criteria or population cohorts for studies never mind the area of interest. However, for research to be useful in changing practice it should reflect the priorities of those who are using the service (Johnston et al., 2008) and issues of relevance.

key concepts in palliative care

176

KEY POINTS

- Research is an important aspect of developing and maintaining high standards of evidence based palliative care.
- There is a wide range of subjects suitable for palliative care research.
- For palliative care research to be successful, it has to address many complex issues: identification of the study population, methodology, ethics, recruitment and attrition.

DISCUSSION

Palliative care research patient population

Borgsteede et al. (2006) examined the consistency with which general practitioners identified palliative care patients if different criteria were used. The GPs were asked to categorise patients from their case load who had recently died against three criteria which are all relevant within palliative care: (1) was the patient receiving non-curative treatment?; (2) was the patient receiving palliative care?; and (3) was the patient's death expected? From the study population 62% were identified as having an expected death, 46% as receiving palliative care and 39% as receiving non-curative treatment. There was some overlap between the groups, but also some patients who were identified in one group but not in others, that is receiving non-curative treatment but not palliative care. These findings have implications for those hoping to recruit to palliative care research as they will need to ensure that their cohort is appropriate to allow the work to be both useful to others in the field, and to identify the correct cohort for the study subject so that the study results are accurate and generalisable to the palliative care population.

Another relevant issue to consider when examining the population being studied within a palliative care study is the potential reluctance of professional staff to use the label 'palliative care' with patients until their physical condition has deteriorated significantly. This may mean that by the time people are acknowledged as requiring palliative care, they may be too ill to participate in any research. On the other hand, research cohorts may be skewed as they only include those who are very unwell with a high symptom burden. The opposite may also apply – that only those patients whose palliative care needs are identified very early in their disease process are included in research as they are well enough to participate. All aspects of this situation mean that the clinicians become the gatekeepers to the research using their clinical judgement about the appropriateness of the individual being approached. Either situation limits the generalisability and usefulness of the research.

Approach/methodology

In order for any research results to be useful, it is vital that the methodology used is appropriate to the subject being studied. Palliative care is a complex subject that may require a variety of different research approaches to address all of the issues identified earlier in this chapter. It is important to remember that, just as effective palliative care delivery is multi-professional, palliative care research may also be multi-professional in nature and examine the topic from a variety of different stances. Randomised controlled trials (RCTs) are not usually seen as a methodology used within palliative care research but Kassa et al. (2006) highlight that palliative care needs more RCTs as most clinical recommendations are based on evidence at level C (consensus/expert opinion) as there is a lack of level A (RCT/meta analysis) and B (non-RCT/cohort studies/case-controlled studies/lower level RCTs) evidence.

Grande and Ingleton (2008) state that a multi-modal approach is appropriate, but requires the researcher to have an understanding of the part that each different methodology can play within the whole research process. Nursing tends to utilise qualitative approaches and while this may be appropriate within the field, there needs to be an assurance that it is undertaken to a high standard. Flemming et al. (2008) undertook a review of six Cochrane Systematic reviews to demonstrate how qualitative approaches can be combined with RCTs to enhance the findings, and highlight that it can be successful with careful planning and experienced researchers.

Ethics

Individuals with palliative care needs are extrinsically and intrinsically vulnerable (Dean and McClement, 2002) and there are conflicting arguments about whether research should be done with this group at all. If we accept that research is necessary to develop the field, then there must be assurances that those participating are protected at all times. This is especially relevant as, with much palliative care research, there is little chance of the research having any direct impact on the care, treatment or prognosis of the participants (Williams, 2007).

All research being undertaken with any client group must receive ethical approval from a local ethics committee. The research question must be relevant, and the methodology and design appropriately rigorous to ensure that the best data can be collected with minimal participant effort. Informed consent is essential and so participants must have the capacity to give it freely (Williams, 2007). Also vital is the right of the participant to withdraw at any time and without giving a reason. The approach should also be flexible enough to be able to respond to the needs of each participant at all times.

Even if the research meets all aspects of ethical approval, if the design is such that the research question cannot be answered at the end of the study, then no-one benefits and participants may have been placed at risk of harm.

Attrition/missing data

Palliative care research will inevitably have a higher attrition rate than research in other areas, and potentially an amount of missing data. If such missing data is non-random (for example – last 48 hours of life), then the results may be biased. The methodology and analysis need to be flexible enough to cope with this and maintain the integrity of the results.

Retrospective data can be collected from next of kin if required, and this may help in identifying unanticipated symptoms which occurred in the last days of life. The researcher needs to ensure that such responses reflect the participant's condition and some aspects are not easy for others to assess, for example, anxiety or distress. Also, patient records may be used, but, again, the participant's perspective is lost.

The researcher needs to address the problems that may be caused by missing data at the start of the study so as to be able to make full use of all the data they are able to obtain.

PRACTICAL APPLICATION OF THE CONCEPT

When she was admitted to the hospice, the staff spent a lot of time with Beth and her family asking them questions, getting to know them and to understand their hopes and fears. After a day, Beth was asked if she would consent to take part in some research the hospice was doing to see how well they were controlling symptoms. Beth was given a leaflet but was too tired to read it. Her family read it. Beth would be asked three times each day to score any symptoms she had and make any comments about her care. The person asking the questions had been a nurse but did not work on the ward. They would pass on any concerns about uncontrolled symptoms to the staff. If Beth didn't want to answer the questions at any time she didn't have to.

Beth's family were concerned it would be too much for her, but she said 'They've been so good to me, and this may help them to be good to others too. This is some good that will come from me dying.'

See also: *patient choice and preferences in palliative care*

FURTHER READING

Addington-Hall, J.M., Bruera, E., Higginson, I.J. and Payne, S. (eds) (2007) *Research Methods in Palliative Care*. Oxford: Oxford University Press.

REFERENCES

Borgsteede, S.D., Deliens, L., Franke, A.L., Willems, D.L., Thm van Eijk, J. and van der Wal, G. (2006) 'Defining the patient population: one of the problems for palliative care research', *Palliative Medicine*, 20: 63–8.

Dean, R.A. and McClement, S.E. (2002) 'Palliative care research: methodological and ethical challenges', *International Journal of Palliative Nursing*, 8(8): 376–80.

Flemming, K., Adamson, J. and Atkin, K. (2008) 'Improving the effectiveness of interventions in palliative care: the potential role of qualitative research in enhancing the evidence from randomised controlled trials', *Palliative Medicine*, 22: 123–31.

research in palliative care

Grande, G. and Ingleton, C. (2008) 'Research in palliative care', in S. Payne, J. Seymour and C. Ingleton (eds), *Palliative Care Nursing. Principles and Evidence for Practice*, 2nd edn. Maidenhead: Open University Press, pp. 625–42.

Johnston, B., Forbat, L. and Hubbard, G. (2008) 'Involving and engaging patients in cancer and palliative care research: workshop presentation', *International Journal of Palliative Nursing*, 14(11): 554–7.

Kassa, S., Hjermstad, M.J. and Loge, J.H. (2006) 'Methodological and structural challenges in palliative care research: how have we fared in the last decade?' *Palliative Medicine*, 20: 727–34.

Perkins, P., Booth, S., Vowler, S.L. and Barclay, S. (2008) 'What are patients' priorities for palliative care research – a questionnaire study', *Palliative Medicine*, 22: 7–12.

Williams, A-L. (2007) 'Recruitment challenges for end-of-life research', *Journal of Hospice and Palliative Nursing*, 9(2): 79–85.

39 resources and information: looking for answers

Jan Woodhouse

DEFINITION

Informational resources are those people and authoritative sources that help patients and their carers to have their questions answered. While verbally answering questions inevitably forms the basis of the information gathered by patients and relatives, there is a place for 'health literacy' (Ache and Wallace, 2009), where reading and numerical skills inform the individuals to function in the healthcare environment.

KEY POINTS

- Patients and carers have a need for information.
- Informational needs change as the disease progresses.
- Written information can enhance understanding.

- Additional measures, such as telephone advice and education programmes, can address informational needs.

DISCUSSION

Informational needs

When someone is diagnosed with an illness it is natural to seek further information about that illness in order to self-manage a response to the threat it poses. When that illness brings the threat of dying and death, then it is not only the patient who might seek extra knowledge but also the family and friends too. Yardley et al. (2009), for example, found that nearly 52% of phone calls to a palliative care advice line came from carers, while the remaining came from healthcare professionals. The NICE guidelines, *Improving Supportive and Palliative Care for Adults with Cancer: The Manual* of 2004, note that information needs to be of a high quality and 'must meet the needs of the target group' adding that it also needs to be 'evidence-based, balanced, and regularly updated' (NICE, 2004: 64). The guidelines go on to point out that service users and experts should be involved in the design and development of information. However, what exactly might the service users, or their carers, want?

Docherty et al. (2008: 167), in their analysis of many papers written on the topic of informational needs of patients and carers, found the following aspects:

- a need to understand the disease, including events that contributed to it and how it might progress;
- need to understand what palliative care is;
- need to know about social welfare aspects, such as benefits;
- need to know about psychological and spiritual care.

As the disease progresses, then additional informational needs emerge such as the issue of pain management. Patients and carers need to understand the timings of drugs, the side effects of drugs and to have an understanding of addiction and tolerance. They may also wish to discuss life-extending therapies. Monterosso et al. (2009) add that carers of children with a terminal illness also need to know about respite care provision plus the parents wished to have information on how to access healthcare professionals.

Hudson et al. (2008: 270) highlight that carers are unprepared for 'the physical, emotional, financial and social impact' that the palliative care stage can bring. As the disease progresses then carers may also need information on the dying process (Hudson et al., 2008) if they have not witnessed death previously.

Patients and carers with less education or who are older have greater informational needs (Docherty et al., 2008). This is further supported by the work of Corli et al. (2009), who showed a decline in an awareness of dying, in relation to the terminal nature of the illness, that appeared to correlate with increasing age. Interestingly they also found that awareness of the potential life-limiting nature of the disease was also linked to the anatomical position of the disease (and here they were looking specifically at cancer). Those who had cancer in the liver or pancreas were more likely to understand that they could die rather than those with breast or skin cancer. Corli et al. (2009) note that while some 67% of patients were aware of their diagnosis, only 58% were aware that their condition was terminal. They comment that psychological factors may account for the discrepancy, such as denial or disavowal. Reading information leaflets may help in counteracting these natural responses to a life-threatening diagnosis.

Enhancing understanding

Docherty et al. (2008) state that when receiving news of such a diagnosis then verbal and written information should be given. Such information should attend to both patients' and carers' information needs. If the carer is having difficulty in coming to terms with the diagnosis then a useful strategy may be to encourage the carer to imagine the feelings of the patient in order to elicit further informational needs. Doherty et al. (2008) recognise that healthcare professionals should provide opportunities for communication and where the patient or carer speaks a different language then to use knowledgeable interpreters. One way of enhancing informational needs is to provide written information in a range of languages.

Ache and Wallace (2009) discuss how written literature for patients and relatives are often poorly designed and beyond the reading ability of many lay people. Written information needs to be written in a language aimed at junior school age – 11 or 12 – using direct language and short paragraphs. The NICE guidelines (2004: 64) also recommend that information is written in a culturally sensitive way and 'composed in plain language'. The print should be greater than a 12-point font (this is especially true for those with visual impairment), avoiding capitalisation of all letters, italics and speciality fonts. There should be ample white space around the short paragraphs and the use of bullet points and boxes are encouraged (Ache and Wallace, 2009). Perhaps there should also be a recommendation to keep a handy stock of information leaflets, or have downloadable copies, as it is in the author's experience that invariably such information ends up being photocopied and then that version is also photocopied, resulting in poor quality reading materials. Materials that are of poor quality may send out a subconscious message that the clinical service being provided is of a similar quality.

Other resources

Hudson et al. (2008) initiated a group education programme, which consisted of three consecutive 1.5 hour weekly sessions for caregivers, that was specifically aimed at giving psychological support to the participants. The group received a guidebook that could prepare the family in supporting the dying relative. The guidebook also contained information on 'problem-solving, positive thinking and relaxation strategies' (Hudson et al., 2008: 272).

As computer ownership increases, then information can be put onto a DVD to allow individuals to peruse a wide range of information or a list of web addresses. The NICE guidelines endorse this by stating that CD-ROMs, DVDs, audio and video cassettes are useful adjuncts to patient leaflets. Macmillan Cancer Care is able to provide a range of CDs that address stages in the cancer journey, including the advanced stage (Macmillan Cancer Care, 2009).

However, it would be wrong to assume that everyone is computer literate or even has the desire to use information technology. It might be an easier option to go along to a local library where there are a plethora of books on specific diseases and narratives that tell of a patient's journey from diagnosis to subsequent death, such as Rachael Clark's book *A Long Walk Home*. Such books usually have lists and contact details of helpful organisations, for example, Macmillan Cancer Care and Age Concern. Macmillan Cancer Care also has information resource services sited within some local libraries.

Yardley et al. (2009) point out that the NICE guidelines set out that specific palliative care information should be available 24 hours a day, 7 days a week and as a consequence hospices are getting used to providing telephone advice for both carers and healthcare professionals.

Who can I turn to?

Monterosso et al.'s (2009) study of children's services found that nurses, including specialist nurses, were predominately the group that families and carers turned to for information, especially in the hospital setting. Local GPs were also regarded as good sources for information, however, this contradicts Docherty et al.'s (2008) study which comments that information was more limited in the community, rather than in other settings. Support from community bodies, such as the church, was also found to be useful.

Hudson et al. (2009) cite that meeting with the family has benefits, where care options and planning can take place and psychological support can be offered. They comment that members of the multi-disciplinary team are available to answer questions raised by the family. At these meetings symptom management, update on the medical condition, discharge planning and the concerns of the carer are often aired. Such meetings have benefited carers by having the opportunity 'to ask questions, debrief and vent feelings' (Hudson et al., 2009: 154) and has improved understanding, dispelling fears as well as providing mediation between family members. As such, this approach may be extremely useful when individual members of a family have found conflicting information.

PRACTICAL APPLICATION OF THE CONCEPT

Edward's sister had just had a diagnosis of breast cancer and the ensuing scans showed that there was significant spread within her body. Edward asked everyone he knew, who might have any knowledge on the topic, for further details. His questions varied, such as 'what is the prognosis?', 'how does the disease spread?', 'if it had been found earlier, would it have prevented the spread?'. After that he scoured bookshops and libraries for specific information on the topic of breast cancer. He got his son to access the internet for additional information but was often perplexed by the medical terminology. Finally he rang Macmillan Cancer Care and ordered a CD about caring for someone with cancer.

See also: *communication; financial aspects for patients and carers; information technology*

FURTHER READING

www.stchristophers.org.uk

REFERENCES

Ache, K.A. and Wallace, L.S. (2009) 'Are end-of-life patient education materials readable?', *Palliative Medicine*, 23: 545–8.

Corli, O., Apolone, G., Pizzuto, M., Cesaris, L., Cozzolino, A., Orsi, L. and Enterri, L. (2009) 'Illness awareness in terminal cancer patients: an Italian study', *Palliative Medicine*, 23: 354–9.

Docherty, A., Owens, A., Asadi-Lari, M., Petchey, R., Williams, J. and Carter, Y.H. (2008) 'Knowledge and information needs of informal caregivers in palliative care: a qualitative systematic review', *Palliative Medicine*, 22: 153–71.

Hudson, P., Quinn, K., Kristjanson, L., Thomas, T., Braithwaite, M., Fisher, J. and Cockayne, M. (2008) 'Evaluation of a psycho-educational group programme for family care givers in home-based palliative care', *Palliative Medicine*, 22: 270–80.

Hudson, P., Thomas, T., Quinn, K. and Aranda, S. (2009) 'Family meetings in palliative care: are they effective?' *Palliative Medicine*, 23: 150–7.

Macmillan Cancer Care (2009) 'Living with and after cancer', available at: www.be.macmillan. org.uk/be/s-187-living-with-and-after-cancer.aspx?ProductTypeFilterID=147, accessed 29 October 2009.

Monterosso, L., Kristjanson, L.J. and Phillips, M.B. (2009) 'The supportive and palliative care needs of Australian families of children who die from cancer', *Palliative Medicine*, 23: 526–36.

National Institute of Clinical Excellence (2004) *Improving Supportive and Palliative Care for Adults with Cancer: The Manual*. London: NICE.

Yardley, S.J., Codling, J., Roberts, D., O'Donnell, V. and Taylor, S. (2009) 'Experiences of 24-hour advice line services: a framework for good practice and meeting NICE guidelines', *International Journal of Palliative Nursing*, 15(6): 266–71.

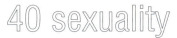

40 sexuality

Moyra A. Baldwin and Jan Woodhouse

DEFINITION

According to Howlett et al. (1997) 'sexuality is much more than the physical sexual act'. For Aylott (2000: 430) it is 'a form of individual expression … cannot be divorced from other human qualities … is not put on hold while an individual is overcoming illness'. From the above we can infer that sexuality still matters when the person has reached the palliative stages of illness, and we can, therefore, assume that sexuality is an essential dimension of palliative care. While the World Health Organisation acknowledges that it is not its official position (WHO, 2002) its website includes a comprehensive definition (see Table 40.1) which clearly states that sexuality is pivotal to being human and is affected by a variety of influences that are a combination of bio-psycho-social factors. Not everyone may be comfortable with this definition. Woodhouse and Baldwin (2008) noted that both patients and healthcare professionals might consider topics such as eroticism and fantasies as taboo. Whether vague or taboo, sexuality is integral to a person's identity and embraced in holistic palliative care.

Table 40.1 WHO (2002) definition of sexuality

Sexuality is a central aspect of being human throughout life and encompasses sex, gender identities and roles, sexual orientation, eroticism, pleasure, intimacy and reproduction. Sexuality is experienced in thoughts, fantasies, desires, beliefs, attitudes, values, behaviour, practices, roles and relationships. While sexuality can include all of these dimensions, not all of them are always experienced or expressed. Sexuality is influenced by the interaction of biological, psychological, social, economic, political, cultural, ethical, legal, historical, religious and spiritual factors.

sexuality

185

KEY POINTS

- Sexuality is an essential aspect of human life.
- Sexuality is difficult to define.
- Expressing sexuality is a component of holistic, psychosocial palliative care.
- There are barriers to exploring patients' sexuality.
- Facilitating patients in expressing sexuality is part of a healthcare professional's role.

DISCUSSION

What does sexuality mean?

Sexuality is a complex issue. It is an essential aspect of human life encompassing self-image, role and relationships, which combine to form a person's social, as well as sexual, identity. Expressing one's sexuality will include aspects relating to body image, reproductive ability, and intimacy. It is not surprising therefore that it can be an emotive and a subjective topic, which may elicit discomfort for both individuals and society. It is value-laden and, according to Jaffe (1977, cited by Cagle and Bolte 2009), a 'double-barreled' taboo sitting alongside mortality: the other taboo inherent in contemporary society, as people will abstain from discussing issues relating to intimacy and sexual contact. Yet these are some of the components of sexuality, others are identified in the WHO (2002) definition above. Clearly sexuality is more than the physical, coital, expression: it is about intimacy, and emotional closeness, which, in the context of palliative care, can create additional psycho-social burdens to those with a life-limiting illness. As with many topics in palliative care, sexuality is both personal and individual and needs to be considered in assessment of patients' bio-psycho-social needs.

Palliative care and meeting sexuality needs

Despite ample literature that encourages healthcare practitioners to offer support and sensitivity to meet individuals' needs in respect of psycho-social issues, culture, ethnicity and sexuality (National Council for Hospices, 1997; NICE 2004; see Woodhouse and Baldwin, 2008, for more detailed exploration), patients' needs remain unmet. Sexuality is recognised by healthcare workers as an important aspect of a patient's holistic and individualised care yet the evidence indicates that there is reluctance on the part of the former to undertake assessments, or care, that enables patients to explore their concerns relating to sexuality.

There are opportunities throughout the care continuum, from the time of diagnosis to palliative care and dying, for healthcare professionals to explore individuals' and families' emotional well-being, their insight, and adaptation to illness. While it may take a mature and, possibly, courageous person to discuss sensitive issues such as sexuality it is important, as Burnard (2000, cited in Woodhouse and Baldwin 2008) rightly notes, for the healthcare professional to be able to recognise and take advantage of opportunities and cues as they arise.

Barriers to facilitating expressing sexuality

Several reasons exist that mitigate healthcare workers facilitating expressing sexuality, for example, they may not see exploring issues relating to sexuality as a priority, especially when compared with more immediate life-threatening, or

Table 40.2   Barriers to facilitating expressing sexuality

Personal

- Embarrassment
- Personal religious beliefs or views
- Not a priority

Organisational

- Focus on medical model of care
- Absence of supervision to discuss issues
- No time

Inter-personal

- No rapport established with the patient

Knowledge/skills (lack of)

- Uncertainty as to when and how to bring up the topic
- Lack of knowledge
- No role model to follow
- Making assumptions

Adapted from Woodhouse and Baldwin (2008).

death, issues. This timidity may be either the healthcare workers' or patients': the former focusing on life-saving care perhaps, and the latter considering issues besides expressing sexuality. Barriers that exist for healthcare professionals facilitating expressing sexuality include personal, organisational, inter-personal and knowledge factors (see Table 40.2).

Assessment

Healthcare professionals working in, or outwith, palliative care use a range of assessment tools when caring for patients with palliative care needs (see Woodhouse and Baldwin, 2008, for examples). The development of personal and professional interactions inherent in the client-professional relationship lends itself to assessing and managing issues of a private and intimate nature such as sexuality. The practitioner's knowledge, skills, attitudes and values will influence how successful assessment will be in eliciting patients' concerns and subsequent management of these concerns in respect of role and expectations (Cort et al., 2004). Assessing sexuality is important but the reluctance by healthcare workers to initiate conversations with patients about their sexuality (Higgins et al., 2006), because they leave it to patients to broach the topic, means that patients' needs will go unrecognised and unmet.

This is where models and frameworks might help, but they can be vague. Assessment needs to include obtaining the patient's health history, comparing the pre-morbid norms with the current state and expression of sexuality (Cort et al., 2004), and the effect both the illness and treatment has had on the individual's perception of his/her sexuality, sexual function, relationships

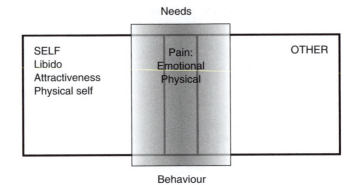

Figure 40.1 *Categories for assessment*

and intimacy. To assess sexuality in palliative care the needs and behaviours of client (self) and partner (other) have to be considered along with the physical self, their libido, and attractiveness (see Figure 40.1).

Use opportunities to discuss sexuality

To help patients, healthcare workers need to look for opportunities to discuss issues of sexuality with patients. Avoiding assumptions, being non-judgemental, and clearly identifying patients' priorities will help to ensure sexual health is addressed. But care is required, what one person considers to be helpful and supportive may be interpreted as prying, inquisitive and 'off-limits' by another. It is essential, therefore, not to make assumptions and to check that the issues to be explored are ones that are important to the person. To facilitate expression of sexuality the practitioner can begin conversation with a question, asking how the illness has affected close relationship with the patient's partner. Starting, however, does require permission and, equally important, privacy (Annon, 1976; Roch and Baldwin, 1998, cited in Woodhouse and Baldwin, 2008). Starting with the least taboo subjects might be helpful (Howlett et al., 1997).

From the knowledge gained the practitioner can advise patients, where relevant, that sexual feelings can change as illness and treatments progress and this might be an opening for sharing more factual information with the patient. The main area, however, is to find out what is important for the patient (Howlett et al., 1997; Woodhouse and Baldwin, 2008). Here the focus is about enabling psycho-social and psycho-sexual adjustment: helping patients optimise interpersonal intimacy and sexual satisfaction.

Sexuality is an aspect of palliative care that can be difficult to address for patients, partners, and health and social care professionals. It is an essential component of palliative care. To provide holistic and individualised care barriers to exploring sexuality need to be overcome so that sexuality and psycho-social adjustment are assessed and managed effectively. Health and social care professionals are in a position to exploit opportunities to facilitate discussion about sexuality with patients and their families. Facilitating expression of sexuality and meeting patients' needs requires health and social care professionals respond proactively and with sensitivity.

PRACTICAL APPLICATION OF THE CONCEPT

Evelyn is 68, had metastatic spread to her right femur, numerous vertebrae and pelvis from a primary breast cancer. She and her husband had been married for 42 years and were described by their daughter as always having had a close, loving relationship. While being nursed in the hospice in the later stages of her illness, she and her husband, Eric, were pleased that the nurse had suggested Eric could stay overnight. Eric and Evelyn declined the offer, which surprised the nurse a little. The relationship the nurse had developed with them was strong enough for Eric to feel able to make an alternative suggestion. Rather than stay overnight what Evelyn, and he, asked for was uninterrupted time in the afternoon when he visited Evelyn.

The nurse agreed with them that she would share this information with her colleagues and that a 'Do Not Disturb' notice would be placed on the door of Evelyn's room when Eric visited in the afternoon. The nurse also reminded them that they could also change their mind if the arrangement for their intimate private time was not meeting their needs.

See also: *communication; holism; patient choice and preferences; reactions of patients and carers*

FURTHER READING

BACUP (2006) *About Sexuality.* Available at: www.macmillan.org.uk/Cancerinformation/Livingwithandaftercancer/Relationshipscommunication/Sexuality/Aboutsexuality.aspx accessed 27 August 2010.

Rice, A.M. (2000a) 'Sexuality in cancer and palliative care 1: effects of disease and treatment', *International Journal of Palliative Nursing*, 6(8): 392–7.

Rice, A.M. (2000b) 'Sexuality in cancer and palliative care 2: exploring the issues', *International Journal of Palliative Nursing*, 6(9): 448–53.

REFERENCES

Aylott, J. (2000) 'Sexuality in care homes: expression or oppression?' *Nursing & Residential Care*, 2(9): 430–35.

Cagle, J.G. and Bolte, S. (2009) 'Sexuality and life-threatening illness: implications for social work and palliative care', *Health & Social Work*, 34(3): 223–32.

Cort, E., Munroe, B. and Olviere, D. (2004) 'Couples in palliative care', *Sexual and Relationship Therapy*, 19(3): 337–54.

Higgins, A., Barker, P. and Begley, C. M. (2006). 'Sexuality: the challenge to espoused holistic care', *International Journal of NursingPractice*, 12: 345–51.

Howlett, C., Swain, M., Fitzmaurice, N., Mountford, K. and Love, P. (1997) 'Sexuality: the neglected component in palliative care', *International Journal of Palliative Nursing*, 3(4): 218–21.

National Council for Hospices and Specialist Palliative Care Services. (1997) 'Feeling better: psychosocial care' in *Specialist Palliative Care*. London. NCHSPCS.

National Institute for Clinical Excellence (2004) *Improving Supportive and Palliative Care for Adults with Cancer*. London. NICE.

Woodhouse, J. & Baldwin, M.A. (2008) 'Dealing sensitively with sexuality in a palliative care context', *British Journal of Community Nursing*, 13(1): 20–5.

World Health Organisation (2002) Gender and Human Rights. Available at: www.who.int/ reproductivehealth/topics/gender_rights/sexual-heal/en/index.html, accessed 12 June 2009.

41 stigma

Elizabeth Mason-Whitehead

DEFINITION

A fundamental prerequisite of the 'human condition' is to notice those people who for whatever reason are in some way 'different' to what we ourselves are or who we are used to. It is within our everyday interactions where we experience difference (Mason-Whitehead and Mason, 2007). Our appreciation of stigma begins at the interface of human contact and this is depicted in Figure 41.1.

There are many descriptions of stigma but this seminal definition provides us with a starting point for our discussion of its association with palliative care;

> While the stranger is present before us, evidence can arise for his possessing an attribute that makes him different from others in the category of persons available, for him to be, and of a less desirable kind – in the extreme a person who is quite thoroughly bad or dangerous, or weak. He is thus reduced in our minds from a whole and usual person to a tainted discounted one. Such an attribute is a stigma. (Goffman, 1963: 53)

Many of us will at some time, whether in our professional or personal lives, be involved with someone who is receiving palliative care. The following paragraphs will prompt us to reflect on our own encounters and how we can both understand and challenge stigma. The subsequent consequences of social exclusion will illuminate a picture of someone who is isolated and alone.

```
┌─────────────────────────────────────────────────────────────────┐
│                                                                   │
│        The Victim(s):  Person(s) ascribed characteristics of difference  │
│                                                                   │
└─────────────────────────────────────────────────────────────────┘

                                   +

┌─────────────────────────────────────────────────────────────────┐
│                                                                   │
│   The Perpetrator(s): Person(s) expressing negativity towards the person(s) │
│               with ascribed characteristics of difference         │
│                                                                   │
└─────────────────────────────────────────────────────────────────┘

                                   =

┌─────────────────────────────────────────────────────────────────┐
│                                                                   │
│        Discrimination and Prejudice: A stigmatising relationship  │
│                                                                   │
└─────────────────────────────────────────────────────────────────┘
```

Figure 41.1   *The interface of a stigmatising relationship*

KEY POINTS

- The impact of stigma can only be fully understood when examined within a cultural context.
- A person who feels stigmatised may endure a number of negative feelings and these are typically isolation, shame and loneliness.
- The disempowerment experienced by stigmatised people may result in them no longer being able to engage with others and this in turn can lead to social exclusion.
- A stigmatised person may present with one or more 'dimensions' of stigma.

DISCUSSION

Our understanding of stigma is indebted to the work of Erving Goffman (1922-82) who in 1963 published *Stigma: Notes on the Management of Spoiled Identity*. His influential work continues to be referenced, re-defined, developed and adapted to fit our ever-changing social world. The work of Jones et al. (1984) builds upon Goffman's contribution and as the following adapted list of the 'Dimensions of Stigma' demonstrates, it focuses our thoughts on how stigma is such a life-changing experience:

1 *Concealability.* How is the condition controllable?
2 *Course.* Does the stigma change as the condition changes over a period of time?
3 *Disruptiveness.* How does the stigma change over time?
4 *Aesthetic.* How does the condition make the person feel about their appearance?
5 *Origin.* Does the person with the condition feel responsible and to blame for their condition?
6 *Peril.* Does the condition present any form of danger and how serious is it?

stigma

191

This discussion considers some of the most significant characteristics of stigma and how this is made apparent when associated with palliative care.

Decision-making: to tell or not to tell?

One of the attributes of people suffering from cancer is that they may have no visible signs of their condition. Goffman (1963) argued that such individuals who had a condition that was 'hidden' or only occasionally became visible were seen as 'discreditable'. Other 'discreditable' conditions include epilepsy where seizures may be infrequent and for much of the time it can be concealed. People with such a diagnoses may find the issue of disclosure difficult because of the fear of being stigmatised. As Scambler (2007) asserts, this can be summarised as to disclose or not to disclose, to tell or not to tell. In the next section we can see how this decision may involve and affect other people.

Family and friends: they can feel stigmatised too

The family and friends of those with a particular condition, understandably, may be very deeply affected and perhaps their feelings and experiences are not always considered. Yet the stigma associated with their loved one's condition may be experienced by themselves too. Goffman (1963) called the 'spread' of stigma to family and friends 'courtesy stigma' and this has been identified in a number of studies. Scambler (2007) argues that where the conditions may have such an impact, then those closest to them will also feel stigmatised. For example, Macdonald's (1988) research into people with rectal cancer, treated with a colostomy, found that nearly half of his participants experienced some kind of stigma. The participants expressed feelings of shame regarding the odour from the stoma and felt they were unclean and some withdrew from day-to-day life. Depending upon the origins and the nature of the cancer, the stigma may be increased and the reason for this are discussed below.

Lifestyle: a culture of blame?

In recent times there has been a focus on the relationship between lifestyle and acquiring a range of medical conditions. The many forms of media, for example, the internet, television, radio, newspapers and magazines, produce articles and news items that show how the risk of acquiring some illnesses can be reduced by changing lifestyle. This shifts the emphasis, from a disease that is acquired through bad luck and chance to a disorder that may be prevented (if, for instance, personal diet and lifestyle are modified). There are now a number of studies that illustrate how people who acquired a 'preventable' cancer have felt stigmatised. For example, a paper by Chapple et al. (2004) showed that people with lung cancer, whether or not they smoked, felt stigmatised because lung cancer is so strongly associated with smoking.

Stigma in the context of social exclusion

An example of understanding stigma in context was in the 1980s, when the human immunodeficiency virus (HIV) was identified particularly with gay men and intravenous drug users. It was during this period where there was little information but considerable fear and gay men (irrespective of their HIV status), in particular, became the victims of attacks, abuse, prejudice and discrimination.

The effect of stigmatising attitudes on individuals and groups can result in prejudice and social exclusion. Social exclusion is often associated with poverty but it is a multidimensional phenomenon that can be best understood in terms of being a result as a catastrophic separation from society (Room, 2005). The experience of social exclusion is to remove an individual's empowerment and therefore the stigmatised person once severed from society finds it difficult to re-engage and participate in the communities where they live.

Challenging stigma and social exclusion

For all of us involved in palliative care, the challenge of working towards overcoming stigma and social exclusion continues to be one of the greatest tests. A number of models have been put forward which consider the roles of individuals and organisations and how they can contribute to reducing stigma within organisations and amongst the general public. Key to this endeavour is delivering correct information about cancer. Education is aimed at dispelling the ignorance that gives rise to the expressions of stigmatisation, for example, the myth that cancer is contagious (Mason et al., 2001).

PRACTICAL APPLICATION OF THE CONCEPT

Anna is a 38-year-old woman with two children of school age, and up until being diagnosed with breast cancer she worked full-time. Anna had always planned her childcare arrangements and was pleased that her children had made such a good relationship with 'Aunty Joyce', a retired lady who collected the children from school and looked after them until Anna returned from work. Anna and Joyce became firm friends. So when Anna found a lump in her breast, Joyce was the first person she told and Anna initially thought that she would be a great source of support for her children. However, on telling Joyce that the tests confirmed that she had breast cancer, Anna noticed a change in Joyce's behaviour; she became more distant, said she could no longer care for the children and stayed away from her house. Anna expressed these concerns to Stephen, her palliative care nurse. Stephen was mindful that cancer is for many people, an illness steeped in ignorance and not spoken about and indeed it may even be known as the 'c' word. Stephen seized the opportunity to speak to Joyce as she left some food outside Anna's door. Joyce's fears were undoubtedly rooted in a lack of knowledge and Stephen was able to provide her with correct information about cancer. Stephen worked with Joyce to overcome her stigma against people with cancer and today she is a valued member of the palliative team who care for Anna and her children.

See also: *attributes of palliative caring; cultural issues; marginalised groups; palliative care for the person with a learning disability; palliative care person with mental ill-health; palliative care education; policy drivers*

FURTHER READING

Green, G. (2009) *The End of Stigma? Changes in the Social Experience of Long Term Illness.* Abingdon: Routledge.
Sontag, S. (1978) *Illness as a Metaphor.* London: Allen Lane.

REFERENCES

Chapple, A., Ziebland, S. and McPherson, A. (2004) 'Stigma, shame and blame experienced by patients with lung cancer: a qualitative study', *British Medical Journal*, 328: 1470 (19 June).
Goffman, E. (1963) *Stigma: Notes on the Management of Spoiled Identity.* London: Penguin.
Jones, E.E., Farina, A., Hastorf, A.H., Markus, H., Miller, D. and Scott, J. (1984) *Social Stigma: The Psychology of Marked Relationships.* New York: Freeman.
Macdonald, L. (1988). 'The experience of stigma: living with rectal cancer', in R. Anderson and M. Bury (eds), *Living with Chronic Illness: The Experience of Patients and their Families.* London: Allen & Unwin.
Mason, T., Carlisle, C., Watkins, C. and Whitehead, E. (eds) (2001) *Stigma and Social Exclusion in Healthcare.* London: Routledge.
Mason-Whitehead, E. and Mason, T. (2007) 'Stigma and exclusion in healthcare settings', In D. Abrams, J. Christian and D. Gordon, (eds), *Multidisciplinary Handbook of Social Exclusion Research.* Chichester: Wiley.
Room, R. (2005) 'Stigma, social inequality and alcohol and drug use', *Drug and Alcohol Review*, 24(2), 143–55.
Scambler, G. (2007) *Sociology as Applied to Medicine.* London: Saunders.

key concepts in palliative care

42 symptom management: complementary and alternative medicine/ integrated health

Joy Parkes and Sue Padmore

DEFINITION

Complementary and Alternative Medicine (CAM) is not easy to define. There is much confusion over these terms which are also known by a variety of other names. Previously, complementary therapies were regarded as an alternative to conventional medicine and the two types were considered mutually exclusive. The concept and application of the terms have evolved over time, as has the position they hold in relation to Conventional Western Medicine. This may itself be considered 'alternative' since Ayurveda and Traditional Chinese Medicine, along with other complete medical systems, are based on traditional principles thousands of years old. On one hand, the term 'alternative' can mean a therapy not provided by Western Medicine, but may also mean a complete independent medical system such as acupuncture which, although alternative to the principles of Western medicine, can be provided within it. The Cochrane Collaboration (2009) defines CAM as 'a broad domain of healing resources that encompasses all health systems, modalities, and practices and their accompanying theories and beliefs, other than those intrinsic to the politically dominant health systems of a particular society or culture in a given historical period'. While this definition is useful, it perpetuates the notion of CAM being outside Western medical practice.

More recently, the term 'complementary' has been applied to those therapies which are used alongside conventional healthcare to provide a comprehensive 'holistic' or 'integrated' approach combining conventional Western medicine with CAM in a 'best of both worlds' approach. From a palliative care perspective, it is interesting to note that both CAM and the hospice movement, sharing similar principles and aims, including person-centeredness

symptom management

195

and quality of life enhancement emerged outside of contemporary Western Medicine. Virtually all hospices now offer an integrated CAM service with approximately 1 in 3 people with cancer using CAM to alleviate disease symptoms or medication side effects (Peace and Manesse, 2002; Chatwin and Tovey, 2004). CAM employs a holistic approach to care rather than being symptom or disease-focused; central to CAM philosophies is personal choice and control for the individual. The fundamental purpose of CAM is to enhance the body's natural healing ability, from a Western Medicine perspective healing means restoration of full physical or psychological health. While restoration to full health is not possible for individuals with life-limiting disease some forms of healing may give comfort and strength.

KEY POINTS

- The use of CAM for symptom management within palliative care is an expanding area.
- Choice and taking control are seen as important reasons for CAM use and should be key to any therapy offered, thereby keeping care person-centred.
- Time, warmth and empathy given by practitioners often correlate with the effectiveness of therapies.
- CAM and palliative care share the holistic approach to care.
- CAM therapies in palliative care are life-enhancing rather than curative.
- There is a clear need for the evidence base for CAM to be enhanced through further funding and research.

DISCUSSION

Aromatherapy, reflexology and massage are consistently reported as the most popular therapies in palliative care (Macmillan Cancer Relief, 2002), although energy healing therapies such as Reiki are becoming increasingly popular (Burden et al., 2005). Nine CAM therapies are identified as useful within supportive and palliative care (Tavares, 2003):

- touch therapies: aromatherapy, massage, reflexology;
- healing/energy therapies: Reiki, spiritual healing, therapeutic touch;
- hypnosis/hypnotherapy;
- acupuncture;
- homeopathy.

These are examples of CAM therapies known to be used in life-limiting situations but are not the only CAM therapies of potential value. Art therapy, diet, herbal modalities, and Indian head massage are utilised and many others are available, the range depending on those therapies in which staff are qualified, and their appropriateness.

CAM practitioners' stance

CAM employs a holistic approach to care, therefore, its role in symptom control is to address the patient's needs more broadly than the contemporary medical pharmacological approach, considering symptoms in context. Treatments are tailored to the recipient's needs at the time. CAM may be delivered to patients, carers, or staff of any age, or stage of their health career; treatments always being 'bespoke'. They can be given at home, in clinics, day centres or hospitals and may well help with the emotional and physical symptoms of cancer, with life-limiting illnesses, or end of life care.

Benefits of CAM

Reduced psychological distress and enhanced symptom control can be seen with the use of aromatherapy when used as an adjunct to orthodox cancer treatments (Dunwoody et al., 2002). Acupuncture and hypnotherapy have been found to reduce pain and nausea (Deng et al., 2004). Acupressure bands may also help relieve the latter. The combined use of reflexology and music therapy has resulted in a reduction of pain, anxiety and feelings of isolation, simultaneously improving communication between patients, families and staff (Magill and Berenson, 2008). CAM can help patients to cope better and to be more relaxed aiding adjustment to their situation. Garnett (2003) purports that trust, warmth and caring by the practitioner are instrumental to this concept. Time expended on treatments is seen as beneficial, boosting self esteem and feelings of well-being.

How CAM works

Health and well-being flow from the harmonious balance of our physical, psychological and spiritual selves: the body, mind and spirit underpin all CAM philosophies. As a corollary, disruption in any of these spheres can impact on the others. Emotional strain may be expressed physically, for example, aches, tension, soreness, skin problems, and digestive upsets. Aims to restore this internal balance are said to stimulate the body's natural self-healing process. In tailoring treatments a CAM practitioner will ask relevant questions about how a person feels, their prevailing symptoms, diet, lifestyle, sleeping patterns, and relationships. This helps the therapist build a 'whole' picture. Patients find it gratifying, therapeutic, in fact, to have the opportunity to talk about themselves.

Risk management and clinical governance

National guidelines were developed on the use of complementary therapies in supportive and palliative care (Tavares, 2003). A review of these guidelines by Hughes and Thomson (2005) found that they had, indeed, been necessary and timely. They had proved a useful tool for the writing of policies, protocols

symptom management

and procedures. Awareness of best practice had been raised, services developed, staff training influenced, all ultimately impacting on quality and safety. Multidisciplinary team-working had improved due to better understanding of therapies. Best practice and commissioning of services were positively affected. These national guidelines along with other key documents such as The House of Lords' Select Committee Report (2000) and the *Guidance on Cancer Services: Improving Supportive and Palliative Care for Adults with Cancer* (National Institute of Clinical Excellence, 2004) have standardised healthcare services, increased the demand for CAM provision and improved clinical governance.

The treatment of cancer may cause side effects such as agitation, anxiety, or sickness and CAM can help alleviate these symptoms. Most complementary therapies, while making the receiver feel mentally stronger and better able to cope, are unlikely to affect medical treatment. Concern, however, has been voiced regarding diet and herbal modalitites regarding issues of safety and interactions with conventional medication. While the medical establishment hails randomised control trials as the gold standard for evidence-based medicine, CAM does not lend itself readily to this method of research. Therefore, choice of research methods must be carefully considered prior to any CAM research. Truly integrated medicine would ensure that all available treatments were accessible to individuals. This model should be embraced to enhance care given to people requiring palliative care, their loved ones and carers. Nurses, in particular, are in a unique position to encompass this model within their role, indeed many nurses working within the palliative care setting are already trained therapists.

PRACTICAL APPLICATION OF CONCEPT

Martha, aged 40, married with two children, was referred to the hospice day care centre by the district nurse. Having undergone a mastectomy for breast cancer, and received radiotherapy and chemotherapy, Martha recovered well and returned to work. Recurring, the disease spread to the bones and Martha, struggling, decided to visit the day care centre. Assessed by the sister-in-charge, given an explanation of the full list of services she and her husband Frank could choose from, Martha was surprised at the range of therapies offered. These included art and craft therapy, acupuncture, physiotherapy, dietary advice, hypnotherapy, reflexology, aromatherapy and Reiki all complementing the full range of nursing and medical services.

Frank declined treatment, but Martha chose aromatherapy and reflexology. Weekly, half-hourly treatments were given each, along with choice of oils, tailored to her feelings and symptoms at the time. Martha reported feeling more relaxed, less anxious, and able to sleep and cope better. Social activities and art therapy also helped. Expressing surprise at how 'lively' and positive the day centre was, Martha resumed work part-time.

All was going well until the cancer spread to her liver and she was admitted to the hospice. Informed of her admission by the Macmillan Nurse, her therapist visited. Suffering anxiety, fatigue, nausea and loss of appetite, Martha chose daily gentle foot massage, Reiki, and vaporised lavender oil in her room. Frank chose massage of his neck and shoulders at her bedside. She died peacefully, Frank receiving support from hospice staff, her children from the art therapist.

See also: *holism; symptom management: common symptoms, difficult/complex symptoms, emergencies, LCP*

FURTHER READING

Hughes, S., and Thomson, A. (2005) *Evaluation of the National Guidelines for the Use of Complementary Therapies in Supportive and Palliative Care*. Available at: www.fih.org.uk, accessed 2 April 2009.

Macmillan Cancer Relief (2002) *Directory of Complementary Therapy Services in UK Cancer Care: Public and Voluntary Sectors*. London: Macmillan Cancer Relief in association with Cambridge publishers.

Tavares, M. (2003) *National Guidelines for the Use of Complementary Therapies in Supportive and Palliative Care*. Available at: www.fih.org.uk, accessed 30 March 2009.

REFERENCES

Burden, B., Herron-Marx, S. and Clifford, C. (2005) 'The increasing use of reiki as a complementary therapy in specialist palliative care', *International Journal of Palliative Nursing*, 11(5): 248–53.

Chatwin, J. and Tovey, P. (2004) 'Complementary and alternative medicine (CAM), cancer and group based action: a critical review of the literature', *European Journal of Cancer Care*, 13: 210–18.

Cochrane Collaboration (2009) 'Complementary and alternative medicine', available at: www.dh.gov.uk, accessed 30 March 2009.

Deng, G., Cassileth, B.R. and Yeung, K.S. (2004) 'Complementary therapies for cancer-related symptoms', *Journal of Supportive Oncology*, 2(5): 419–26.

Dunwoody, L., Smyth, A. and Davidson, R. (2002) 'Cancer patients' experiences and evaluations of aromatherapy massage in palliative care', *International Journal of Palliative Nursing*, 8(10): 497–504.

Garnett, M. (2003) 'Sustaining the cocoon: the emotional inoculation produced by complementary therapies in palliative care', *European Journal of Cancer Care*, 12: 129–36.

House of Lords Select Committee on Science and Technology (2000) *Complementary and Alternative Medicine: Session 1999–2000*, 6th Report. Available at: www.dh.gov.uk, accessed 30 March 2009.

Hughes, S. and Thomson, A. (2005) *Evaluation of the National Guidelines for the Use of Complementary Therapies in Supportive and Palliative Care*. Available at: www.fih.org.uk, accessed 2 April 2009.

Macmillan Cancer Relief (2002) *Directory of Complementary Therapy Services in UK Cancer Care: Public and Voluntary Sectors*. London: Macmillan Cancer Relief in association with Cambridge publishers.

Magill, L. and Berenson, S. (2008) 'The conjoint use of music therapy and reflexology with hospitalized advanced stage cancer patients and their families', *Palliative and Supportive Care*, 6(3): 289–96.

National Institute for Clinical Excellence (2004) *Guidance on Cancer Services: Improving Supportive and Palliative Care for Adults with Cancer: The Manual*. Available at: http://www.nice.org.uk, accessed 1 April 2009.

Peace, G. and Manesse, A. (2002) 'The Cavendish Centre for integrated cancer care: assessment of patient needs and responses', *Complementary Therapy Medicine*, 10(1): 33–41.

Tavares, M. (2003) *National Guidelines for the Use of Complementary Therapies in Supportive and Palliative Care*. Available at: www.fih.org.uk, accessed 30 March 2009.

43 symptom management: common symptoms

Catherine Black

DEFINITION

The World Health Organisation's (2002) definition of palliative care highlights that the control of pain and other distressing symptoms is a major tenet of high quality care. Within the United Kingdom, control of symptoms is one of the gold standards for palliative care within community settings. Many authors (Edmonds, 2004a; Faull, 2005; Hill, 2006) highlight the vital role that managing individual symptoms plays within palliative care. All members of the team need to recognise that, unless physical symptoms are managed appropriately, the individual cannot possibly begin to address other 'higher level' issues such as what their illness means to them and preparing themselves and their families for the future. Therefore, managing physical symptoms should not been seen as basic care – but should be seen as the vital underpinning care upon which all high-quality palliative care is based.

Hill (2006: 40) defines symptoms as 'the problems a patient presents'. This definition is important as carers need to recognise that each individual will find different problems more difficult to manage and cope with, and that professionals need to work with each person to prioritise their problems appropriately. This can only be done by accurate, in-depth and regular assessment of each symptom, using appropriate tools where available. Potential causes of each symptom need to be identified and, where appropriate for the individual, investigations carried out to confirm the cause (Edmonds, 2004a). This is vital, as many symptoms have several potential causes, but the cause may have implications for the best treatment to use. There also needs to be an awareness of the inter-relationship between different symptoms and their treatments (Kinley, 2005), for example, pain can cause nausea; opiates can cause constipation which, in turn, can cause nausea, and so while each symptom must be assessed and managed individually, the team must also always be aware of the holistic presentation (Edmonds, 2004a).

The team also needs to be aware that there are limitations to symptom control and not all symptoms can be managed successfully all of the time (Faull, 2005). In such cases the team needs to work towards a solution that is acceptable to the individual, and manages the distress caused by the symptom as well as the symptom itself.

KEY POINTS

- Management of physical symptoms is key within palliative care.
- Accurate and regular assessment is vital in order to manage symptoms.
- Assessment should include both the individual symptoms and an holistic overview to check for inter-relationships between symptoms.
- Medication is a primary treatment of the majority of physiological symptoms and needs careful adjustment to ensure the best drug and dose is used for the individual.

DISCUSSION

Kinley (2005) identified that some of the most common symptoms in advanced illness are pain, nausea and vomiting, dyspnoea and constipation.

Pain

Black (2009) outlined the prevalence of pain as a symptom within several life limiting conditions and across the conditions the occurrence of pain ranged from 25–96% of patients. In all conditions, the occurrence and severity of pain experienced increased with disease progression. For patients, pain is the most feared symptom and is often associated with progression in disease and worsening of prognosis (Black et al., 2007). Black et al. (2007) undertook a literature review of pain assessment tools. They highlighted a range of assessment tools that can be used, but stressed that no tool will suit all patients, and that no tool is a replacement for good communication between the patient and the professional assessing them.

While the holistic nature of pain must not be underestimated, pharmacological management is required for the majority of individuals after assessment.

The WHO 3 step analgesic ladder (Black, 2009) is the basis for managing all types of pain. The underpinning principles are that drugs are given: by mouth, by the clock, by the ladder, for the individual and there is attention to detail. The ladder outlines how to progressively increase analgesia incrementally from non-opioids to strong opioids. It must be recognised that the starting point will depend on the pain assessment, and that individuals may be required to commence on strong opioids without working through the ladder if their pain is severe. Adjuvant medication also has an important role in managing pain. This includes corticosteroids, tricyclic antidepressants and anticonvulsants.

Nausea and vomiting

Nausea and vomiting is a symptom of advanced cancer and other long-term conditions, such as heart failure and lung conditions (Perkins and Dorman, 2009). The main treatment is with drugs (Pace, 2004; Kinley, 2005), but anti-emetics are often under-prescribed (Glare et al., 2008). Potential causes of nausea are wide-ranging and include strong smells, drugs, raised intra-cranial pressure, constipation, severe pain and electrolytes imbalance (Kinley, 2005) and so a range of investigations may need to be undertaken, if the patient's condition allows. These should include blood tests of electrolytes and renal function (Pace, 2004). If the patient is too frail then decisions can be made on clinical grounds. If the causes of the nausea and vomiting can be reversed (e.g. hypercalcaemia), this is the best form of management, and current medication should be reviewed and drugs causing nausea discontinued if possible.

Anti-emetics have different modes of action, and should be chosen to be suitable for the assessed cause. They need to be given at an appropriate dose and via an appropriate route, either parentally or rectally in a vomiting patient. If the first choice of anti-emetic is not successful in 24 hours then the dose should be changed or another anti-emetic added. If a second anti-emetic is added, then it should have different mode of action to the first.

Dyspnoea

Dyspnoea (breathlessness) is a common symptom in advanced illness and one that has a detrimental impact on quality of life (Jennings et al., 2009). There are many physiological causes, for example, anaemia, fluid overload, chest infection, pleural effusion, and these should be investigated and treated wherever possible. However, there is a large psychological impact and cause of dyspnoea, for example, anxiety and fear, and such factors must be considered in an assessment. Maher and Hemming (2005) outline several assessment tools for dyspnoea, but do highlight that all of the tools are limited in their ability to undertake a holistic assessment.

The use of oxygen in patients with dyspnoea who are not hypoxic is not supported by research evidence (Edmonds, 2004b), but it is seen as having an important psychological benefit for the individual. This is important but needs to be assessed against the potential restrictions in mobility and socialising created by the use of oxygen (Maher and Hemming, 2005). Although the numbers in studies are small, there is evidence to support the use of oral or subcutaneous opioids for dyspnoea, but not for the use of nebulised (inhaled) opioids (Jennings et al., 2009).

There is research evidence that teaching the individual breathing control and relaxation can help to improve their dyspnoea (Edmonds, 2004b). Such techniques can be taught by any appropriate member of the team (nurse, physiotherapist, occupational therapist), but should then be supported and used consistently by the multidisciplinary team as a whole.

Constipation

Constipation is a common symptom in palliative care. Some 90% of patients taking opioids have some degree of constipation, and 60% of palliative care patients who are not taking opioids also have constipation to some level (Sykes, 2004). Aperients are the main management of constipation, and should be used prophylactically for all patients on opioids. The individual can also make changes to life style and diet, which can be helpful (Miles et al., 2009).

As with the management of other symptoms discussed, there are a variety of medications that can be used, each of which has a different method of action. However, a recent Cochrane review (Miles et al., 2009) concluded that there is a lack of evidence to support the use of any particular laxative and indeed the studies showed that all laxatives are ineffective for a number of patients. Laxatives may be combined but, again, there is little evidence to support any particular combination.

PRACTICAL APPLICATION OF THE CONCEPT

Joe was admitted with nausea and vomiting. His GP had prescribed anti-emetics the day before, but Joe was unable to tolerate them orally. On admission he was drowsy, dehydrated and had a distended abdomen.

When talking to the doctor, Joe stated that his back pain had been getting worse and he had increased his use of 'as required' liquid morphine at home five days ago. This increase in dose coincided with his nausea. On questioning Joe also stated that he hadn't had his bowels opened for four days but he put this down to not eating and drinking as much as usual. He hadn't been taking his laxatives while he felt nauseous.

Joe was discharged after seven days. His analgesia had been re-titrated and the dose increased appropriately, his anti-emetics had been changed and the importance of taking his laxatives regularly had been reinforced. He was invited to a day unit on a weekly basis so that his symptoms could be monitored and his medication adjusted as required.

See also: holism; symptom management: complementary and alternative medicine, difficult/ complex symptoms, emergencies, LCP

FURTHER READING

Doyle. D., Hanks, G. and Macdonald, N. (eds) (2004) *The Oxford Textbook of Palliative Medicine*, 3rd edn. Oxford: Oxford University Press.
www.palliativedrugs.com

REFERENCES

Black, C. (2009) 'Pharmacological management of pain in palliative care', *International Journal of Disability and Human Development*, 8(1): 3–8.

Black, C., Aveyard, B., Smith, P. and Schofield, P. (2007) 'Pain assessment in terminal cancer', *Journal of Community Nursing*, 21(5): 19–21.

Edmonds, P. (2004a) 'Symptom assessment', in N. Sykes, P. Edmonds and J Wiles, (eds), *Management of Advanced Disease*, 4th edn. London: Arnold Publishers, pp. 51–4.

Edmonds, P. (2004b) 'Breathlessness', in N. Sykes, P. Edmonds and J. Wiles (eds), *Management of Advanced Disease*, 4th edn. London: Arnold Publishers, pp. 73–82.

Faull, C. (2005) 'The context and principles of palliative care' in C. Faull, Y. Carter and L. Daniels, (eds), *Handbook of Palliative Care*, 2nd edn. Oxford: Blackwell Publishing, pp. 1–21.

Glare. P., Dunwoodie, D., Clark, K., Ward, A., Yates, P., Ryan, S. and Hardy, J. (2008) 'Treatment of nausea and vomiting in terminally ill cancer patients', *Drugs*, 68(18): 2575–90.

Hill, S. (2006) 'Symptom management: a framework', in J. Cooper (ed), *Stepping Into Palliative Care 2*. Oxford: Radcliffe Publishing, pp. 40–76.

Jennings, A.L., Davies, A.N., Higgins, J.P.T., Broadley, K.E. and Anzures-Cabrera, J. (2009) 'Opioids for the palliation of breathlessness in terminal illness (review)', *The Cochrane Collaboration*, Issue 3.

Kinley, J. (2005) 'Controlling nausea and vomiting in palliative care patients', *Nurse Prescribing*, 3(4): 141–50.

Maher, D. and Hemming, L. (2005) 'Palliative care for breathless patients in the community', *British Journal of Community Nursing*, 10(9): 414–18.

Miles, C., Fellowes, D., Goodman, M.L. and Wilkinson, S.S.M. (2009) 'Laxatives for the management of constipation in palliative care patients (review)', *The Cochrane Collaboration*, Issue 3.

Pace, V. (2004) 'Nausea and vomiting', in N. Sykes, P., Edmonds and J. Wiles, (eds), *Management of Advanced Disease*, 4th edn. London: Arnold Publishers, pp. 156–67.

Perkins, P. and Dorman, S. (2009) 'Haloperidol for the treatment of nausea and vomiting in palliative care patients (review)', *The Cochrane Collaboration*, Issue 3.

Sykes N. (2004) 'Constipation and diarrhoea', in N. Sykes, P. Edmonds and J. Wiles (eds), *Management of Advanced Disease*, 4th edn. London: Arnold Publishers, pp. 94–100.

World Health Organisation (2002) Definition. Available at: www.who.int/cancer/palliative/ definition/ accessed 12 June 2009.

key concepts in palliative care

44 symptom management: difficult/ complex symptoms

Catherine Black

DEFINITION

It is challenging to define what a 'difficult' or 'complex' symptom is within the field of palliative care. In their study, Blomberg and Sahlberg-Blom (2007) did not even try to develop a definition. They simply asked staff to identify and talk about 'difficult problems', and all problems that the staff subsequently identified as difficult were accepted as such. Corner (2008) challenged such an approach by highlighting that most of the research undertaken into difficult and complex symptoms is by clinicians, and so could have an underpinning biomedical stance. Also, such work will often highlight the symptoms that are seen as complex by those undertaking the research, with little emphasis on those that the patient and family see as complex and difficult. For these reasons, all relevant perspectives need to be included.

This chapter will not attempt to identify difficult and complex symptoms and discuss their management, but will instead look at the underpinning reasons why a symptom may be labelled as difficult. This can be from several different perspectives – patient, family and professional carers.

KEY POINTS

- All symptoms in end of life care are multi-factorial in nature with physical, psychological, social and spiritual elements.
- Professionals may see a symptom as 'manageable' but this may not mean that the patient and family do not see it as 'difficult'.
- Any symptom can become labelled as difficult or complex if the team managing it do not have access to the knowledge, skills and equipment required to do this successfully.

DISCUSSION

Cicely Saunders first described the multi-factorial nature of symptoms, within palliative care, in 1969 (Greenstreet, 2001) when she outlined the concept of 'total pain'. Pain was described as having four components: physical, psychological, social and spiritual. Each of these needed to be managed successfully in order for the pain experience to be alleviated. This model can be applied to many of the symptoms seen in palliative care as they may have many causes, not all of which will be physical. Indeed, to manage symptoms successfully, we need to be aware of non-physical causes and not be limited to approaching symptom management from a purely physical perspective.

Care of the dying includes many dimensions of suffering, and not all of these may be alleviated (Blomberg and Sahlberg-Blom, 2007) on all occasions. While removal of a symptom may be seen as successful management, professionals must acknowledge that this does not necessarily make that symptom any less of a concern to the patient (Corner, 2008). If we consider all of the components identified by Saunders (Greenstreet, 2001), we can see that simply managing only the physical causes, and maybe reducing the symptom itself, may not relieve the consequences associated with the symptom – such as fear and anxiety relating to the risk of the symptom returning.

Any symptom can be labelled as difficult – even those that may be seen as common. There will always be situations where individual symptoms cannot be managed successfully and in this circumstance it will be labelled as 'difficult' by some, or all, of those involved. When symptoms are labelled as difficult by the patient, family or the professionals, we should take the time to consider in what way it is difficult: Is it difficult to watch? Difficult to bear? Cannot be controlled? Difficult to manage? Or is there a significant meaning of the symptom for some of those involved? (Corner, 2008). For the patient with cancer, the knowledge that their pain may be a sign that their cancer is spreading may increase the spiritual, psychological and social aspects of their pain experience. Therefore, even though physiologically their disease has not progressed, their pain experience may increase as the other factors become increasingly important. For the relative who has seen this symptom before in other loved ones, it may be a reminder of previous bereavement and a confirmation of a denied prognosis.

Extreme breathlessness is a difficult symptom to watch, especially when accompanied by fear and anxiety (Corner, 2008). Breathing is such a fundamental and necessary part of living, that we only notice it in others when they are having problems. Once the observer becomes aware of the problem, then their anxiety is raised also – and difficulties with breathing are hard to disguise from onlookers in a way that pain is not. Blomberg and Sahlberg-Blom (2007) found that in such situations, the professional carers may use 'closeness' and 'distance' to balance their relationship with the patient in order to protect themselves. They may prioritise physical tasks and routine care rather than becoming involved in more psycho-social aspects that may be required. They highlight that teamwork is the key to managing difficult symptoms and situations and to prevent stress and burnout amongst staff, and so ensuring that optimal care is delivered focusing on all potential causes and implications of symptoms.

Some symptoms may be labelled as difficult in certain circumstances because they cannot be managed in that particular setting. This may be due to organisational structures and constraints preventing the use of certain symptom management techniques (Tishelman et al., 2004). Specialist palliative care areas may receive referrals from non-specialist areas for patients with 'difficult' symptoms, only to find on admitting the patient, that with their knowledge and skills they find they can manage the symptom relatively easily. This can lead to the specialist area under-estimating their own expertise and labelling the care given in other areas as sub-standard. This fails to recognise the organisational constraints that colleagues in other settings may be working under. These may include difficulty accessing syringe drivers or anxiety about prescribing and administering opiates, but will have an impact on their ability to successfully manage the symptom. Lorenz et al. (2004) highlight the opposite situation where palliative patients are receiving treatment specialised to the area where they are currently being cared for, for example palliative chemotherapy, and such treatment would make it difficult for them to be cared for in a hospice, and so they are denied admission. Both examples show that location can have an impact on whether a symptom is seen as difficult.

The social aspects of the family's role in the management of symptoms cannot be overstated. Beckstrand et al. (2009) asked oncology nurses to identify obstacles that prevented them giving appropriate end of life care. Eight of the top ten obstacles related to family attitudes and behaviours. This included angry family members, anxiety among family members, unrealistic views of prognosis, and family members imposing their wishes on the management of symptoms. Examples of this may include family members requesting that patients receive more analgesia when the patients themselves refuse it, or the family requesting that patients receives less analgesia as they appear too sedated. Both situations may lead to sub-optimal management of the patient's pain from the professional or family perspective, and so the pain becomes labelled as difficult. This, in turn, will create more anxiety and stress in an already challenging situation.

Patients, relatives and professionals fear symptoms that cannot be controlled and managed. Corner (2008) suggests that we need to examine the reasons why the problem is difficult so that we can identify what can be changed. All members of the team, including patients and relatives, need to be involved in this process so that all of the elements influencing the problem can be identified. Only by viewing each problem holistically, from all perspectives, will we begin to get close to ensuring symptom-free end of life care.

PRACTICAL APPLICATION OF THE CONCEPT

I was attending a pain management clinic as a post-registration oncology student when I recognised the next patient the consultant was due to see. Mr Harding had been re-referred to the clinic three months earlier with recurrence of severe back pain that hadn't been managed with analgesics. A review of his referral letter showed that, at the time of his original referral (18 months ago), his wife was being treated for cancer at the oncology hospital where I had worked. He had successfully responded to acupuncture at that time.

As the consultant placed the acupuncture needles and talked to Mr Harding, he asked about his wife. Mr Harding began to cry and explained that his wife had died suddenly and unexpectedly four months ago. The consultant offered his condolences and I offered to stay with Mr Harding. He described how his wife had died, in hospital, after a sudden deterioration. She had been admitted for an overnight blood transfusion and her death was a shock for him and his adult daughter. He felt unable to cope without his wife. He was unable to touch any of her things – the hair brush that she left on the kitchen table as she was leaving the house to be admitted was still where she left it. His back pain had recurred within days of her death and he could find no physical reason for it.

I talked with Mr Harding for over an hour, and passed the information to the consultant. We discussed Mr Harding's back pain in the light of this information as a 'total pain' with psychological and spiritual elements, and potential changes that may be made to his management, including referral to other members of team, including a psychologist.

See also: *holism*

FURTHER READING

Doyle, D., Hanks, G. and Macdonald, N. (eds) (2004) *The Oxford Textbook of Palliative Medicine*, 3rd edn. Oxford: Oxford University Press.

REFERENCES

Beckstrand, R.L., Moore, J., Callister, L. and Bond, A.E. (2009) 'Oncology nurses' perceptions of obstacles and supportive behaviours at the end of life', *Oncology Nursing Forum*, 36(4): 446–53.

Blomberg, K. and Sahlberg-Blom, E. (2007) 'Closeness and distance: a way of handling difficult situations in daily care', *Journal of Clinical Nursing*, 16: 244–54.

Corner, J. (2008) 'Working with difficult symptoms', in S. Payne, J. Seymour and C. Ingleton (eds), *Palliative Care Nursing: Principles and Evidence for Practice*, 2nd edn. Maidenhead: Open University Press, pp. 241–59.

Greenstreet, W. (2001) 'The concept of total pain: a focused patient care study', *British Journal of Nursing*, 10(19): 1248–55.

Lorenz, K.A., Asch, S.M., Rosenfeld, K.E., Hui Lui, M.S. and Ettner, S.L. (2004) 'Hospice admission practices: where does hospice fit in the continuum of care?', *Journal of the American Geriatrics Society*, 52: 725–30.

Tishelman, C., Bernhardson, B-M., Blomberg, K., Börjeson, S., Franklin, L., Johansson, E., Leveälahti, H., Sahlberg-Blom, E. and Ternestedt, B-M. (2004) 'Complexity in caring for patients with advanced cancer', *Journal of Advanced Nursing*, 45(4): 420–9.

45 symptom management: emergencies

Catherine Black

DEFINITION

Emergencies in palliative care in patients with advanced disease are common (Forrest and Napier, 2006). This chapter will focus on physical emergencies, and the most common of these are spinal cord compression, superior vena cava obstruction and hypercalcaemia (Rosser, 2007a), and malignant bowel obstruction (Lynch and Sarazine, 2006). Such conditions can have a detrimental impact on the individual's function and quality of life (Barton, 2005), and prompt recognition and appropriate management can help to minimise the permanent effects (Rosser, 2007a). If not appropriately managed, such emergencies may also lead to the individual's death.

Whether an event is classified as an emergency will depend upon the clinical situation of the patient and the type of event occurring. For example, the development of early spinal cord compression in an individual with a slow growing tumour is an emergency, but in a patient already bedridden from extensive metastases and rapidly progressing disease, it is not. Also, it is imperative that the patient's current physical condition and their ability to undergo treatment are considered. For example the patient may have to be transferred to another hospital to have radiotherapy, and it must be considered if they can cope with such a transfer. If interventions are seen as inappropriate, then the team must communicate with the patient and family to fully explain the situation, and reduce stress by pre-empting expected changes and proactively managing further symptoms (Forrest and Napier, 2006).

- Whether an event is classified as an emergency requiring emergency treatment will depend on the clinical situation of the individual.
- Rapid assessment and initiation of appropriate treatment are key to minimising permanent disabilities and preventing mortality.
- Some emergencies can be predicted as likely in certain patient groups, and such patients must be informed of the signs and symptoms and actions they should take, for example contact numbers.

DISCUSSION

Spinal cord compression (SCC)

Warnock et al. (2008) discuss that SCC can occur in up to 5% of patients with cancer, although Rosser (2007a) states that occurrence is up to 10% in this group. It is most common in cancer of the breast, lung or prostate. In the majority of cases, SCC develops when a metastases in a vertebral body extends into the epidural space and compresses the spinal cord leading to ischemia and permanent neurological deficit below the damaged area (Barton, 2005; Rosser, 2007a; Drudge-Coates and Rajbabu, 2008a).

Early symptoms are varied in type and severity and therefore hard to detect. Drudge-Coates and Rajbabu (2008a) identify pain, weakness, sensory deficit and autonomic dysfunction as the main symptoms. There can also be numbness or tingling in the lower limbs. Later symptoms include loss of mobility, and altered bladder and bowel function (Rosser, 2007a; Warnock et al., 2008).

Rapid diagnosis is vital as outcomes after treatment are related to the amount of disability presented initially, as the damage to the spinal cord is progressive and irreversible. Only 5–10% of patients who have lost the ability to walk by presentation will regain it after treatment (Rosser, 2007a). It is therefore imperative that patients at risk of developing SCC are made aware of that potential and the symptoms they should be aware of so that they can seek help urgently (NICE, 2008). Patients with known cancer reporting such symptoms should be treated as having SCC until proven otherwise.

Treatment is often high dose steroids and radiotherapy. These treatments may take several days to relieve all the symptoms fully (Drudge-Coates and Rajbabu, 2008b). Surgical decompression may be an option, depending on the ability of the patient to undergo the procedure, and is the only treatment that will relieve the decompression immediately. Most patients will have a change in their functional ability following SCC, and will require a period of rehabilitation and adjustment. The entire multi-disciplinary team will be involved, and careful preparation will be required before discharge home.

Superior vena cava obstruction (SVCO)

SVCO describes a condition where blood flow through the superior vena cava is obstructed. In 80% of cases cancer is the underlying cause, and in 50%

of these cases SVCO the presenting symptom of that cancer (Barton, 2005; Forrest and Napier, 2006).

Development of SVCO may be gradual, but eventually the patient presents with increasing dyspnoea. On examination there will be distension of neck and chest veins, swelling of face and arms, and stridor (Harris et al., 2004; Barton, 2005; Rosser, 2007a). Symptoms may worsen when the patient bends forwards or lies down.

Treatment of the cause of the obstruction will depend on the patient's condition. Chemotherapy or radiotherapy to shrink the tumour may be an option depending on the histology of the tumour (Rosser, 2007b). Insertion of a stent may lead to a rapid resolution of symptoms and is a well-tolerated procedure (Harris et al., 2004). Symptomatic treatment of dyspnoea will also be required. Psychological support for the patient and family will be needed to manage the anxiety of the situation.

Hypercalcaemia

Hypercalcaemia is corrected serum calcium of over 2.6 mmol/l (Rosser, 2007a) and is after the calcium level is adjusted for the level of albumin in the blood. It is the commonest metabolic disorder in cancer patients occurring in up to 30% of this group (Forrest and Napier, 2006). It is most common in those with cancers of the breast, lung, head and neck, renal tumours, myeloma and lymphoma (Rosser, 2007a) and is more common in patients with bone metastases, but can occur without their presence.

The development of hypercalcaemia is a poor prognostic indictor with median survival after it's diagnosis of three months (Davies, 2004), although 50% of patients die within thirty days (Forrest and Napier, 2006).

Initial symptoms include thirst, dehydration, nausea and constipation (Davies, 2004; Forrest and Napier, 2006) and hypercalcaemia should always be suspected in patients with known bone metastases. There is a debate about whether greater degrees of hypercalcaemia lead to an increase in the severity of symptoms (Davies, 2004; Forrest and Napier, 2006), but without treatment, symptoms can develop to include confusion, psychosis and cardiac arrhythmias and coma.

Initial treatment is to rehydrate the patient by both encouraging oral fluids and commencing an intra-venous infusion (IVI) (Rosser, 2007b). Intravenous bisphosphonates can also be commenced. These inhibit bone resorption and have a rapid action to reduce serum calcium and symptoms, although it may take seven to ten days for serum calcium to reach its lowest level (Barton, 2005). IV bisphosphonates can then be given for maintenance treatment and this can often take place on an out-patient basis.

Bowel obstruction

Bowel obstruction occurs when the normal functioning of the bowel is stopped or reduced by a narrowing of the bowel lumen (Lynch and Sarazine, 2006). It may be caused by tumour growth, radiotherapy or surgical adhesions, and is commonest in patients in the advanced stages of abdominal cancers (Letizia and Norton, 2003).

Presenting symptoms will vary depending on which area of the bowel is obstructed but generally include large volume vomits, nausea which may be relieved by vomiting, lack of passing of faeces, abdominal distension, bowel sounds may be increased or absent, and abdominal pain (Chiltern and Faull, 2005).

If the patient is well enough, surgical intervention may be an option for treatment. Non-surgical options include resting the bowel by use of a naso-gastric tube and maintaining the patient nil by mouth with an IVI to maintain hydration. Drugs that increase gastric peristalsis such as metoclopramide and stimulant laxatives must be discontinued as they could worsen the condition (Chiltern and Faull, 2005). Pain and nausea can be managed with medication but the oral route must not be used (Letizia and Norton, 2003). Hyoscine butylbromide will help to control secretions and so help to manage colicky pain and nausea.

PRACTICAL APPLICATION OF THE CONCEPT

Mr James phoned his GP on Monday morning. He had been diagnosed with cancer of the prostate three weeks earlier, but since Friday evening he had increasing pins and needles in his legs and this morning he was struggling to stand, and couldn't pass urine. The GP arranged urgent admission to the local hospital, and after assessment when spinal cord compression was diagnosed, Mr James was transferred to the regional cancer centre for treatment of steroids and radiotherapy.

Two weeks later Mr James was transferred to the local hospice for rehabilitation. He could not stand and so was using a wheelchair. He also had a urinary catheter in situ. It was a further 12 weeks before Mr James was discharged home as his functional ability did not increase and major readjustments had to be made to the house to accommodate the wheelchair. Mr James became depressed and withdrawn and his wife had difficulty coping with her new role as a carer.

Mr James lived for a further two years after his SCC. During this time he had regular admissions to the hospice for respite care, and increasing admissions to the hospital for management of problems caused by his lack of mobility.

See also: *holism; multi-disciplinary teams*

FURTHER READING

Doyle, D., Hanks, G. and Macdonald, N. (eds) (2004) *The Oxford Textbook of Palliative Medicine*, 3rd edn. Oxford: Oxford University Press.

REFERENCES

Barton, R. (2005) 'Managing complications of cancer' in C. Faull, Y. Carter and L. Daniels (eds), *Handbook of Palliative Care*, 2nd edn. Oxford: Blackwell Publishing, pp. 208–39.

Chiltern, A. and Faull, C. (2005) 'The management of gastrointestinal symptoms and advanced liver disease', in C. Faull, Y. Carter and L. Daniels (eds), *Handbook of Palliative Care*, 2nd edn. Oxford: Blackwell Publishing, pp.150–84.

Davies, A.N. (2004) 'Hypercalcaemia and hyponatraemia', in N. Sykes, P. Edmonds and
    J. Wiles (eds), *Management of Advanced Disease*, 4th edn. London: Arnold Publishers,
    pp. 270–9.

Drudge-Coates, L. and Rajbabu, K. (2008a) 'Diagnosis and management of malignant spinal
    cord compression: part 1', *International Journal of Palliative Nursing*, 14(3): 110–16.

Drudge-Coates, L. and Rajbabu, K. (2008b) 'Diagnosis and management of malignant spinal
    cord compression: part 2', *International Journal of Palliative Nursing*, 14(4): 175–80.

Forrest, J. and Napier, M. (2006) 'Emergencies in palliative care', in J. Cooper (ed.), *Stepping
    into Palliative Care 2*. Oxford: Radcliffe Publishing, pp. 130–47.

Harris, S., Brown, E., Irvine, A. and O'Dowd, J. (2004) 'Superior vena cava obstruction and
    spinal cord compression', in N. Sykes, P. Edmonds and J. Wiles (eds), *Management of
    Advanced Disease*, 4th edn. London: Arnold Publishers, pp. 251–61.

Letizia, M. and Norton, E. (2003) 'Successful management of malignant bowel obstruction',
    Journal of Hospice and Palliative Nursing, 5(3): 152–8.

Lynch, B., and Sarazine, J. (2006) 'A guide to understanding malignant bowel obstruction',
    International Journal of Palliative Nursing, 12(4): 164–71.

National Institute for Health and Clinical Excellence (NICE) (2008) *Metastatic Spinal Cord
    Compression: Diagnosis and Management of Adults at Risk of and with Metastatic Spinal
    Cord Compression*. London: NICE.

Rosser, M. (2007a) 'Palliative care emergencies 1: Diagnosis', *Nursing Times*, 103(33): 28–9.

Rosser, M. (2007b) 'Palliative care emergencies 2: Management', *Nursing Times*, 103(34): 26–7.

Warnock, C., Cafferty, C., Hodson, S., Kirkham, E., Osguthorpe, C., Siddall, J., Walsh, R. and
    Foran, B. (2008) 'Evaluating the care of patients with malignant spinal cord compression
    at a regional cancer centre', *International Journal of Palliative Nursing*, 14(10): 510–15.

46 symptom management: the liverpool care pathway for the dying patient (LCP)

Richard Latten, John Ellershaw and Deborah Murphy

DEFINITION

Care of patients during the dying phase of their illness is a key area of palliative
care. While good quality care of the dying shares many principles of good
quality palliative care in general, such as symptom control, psychological support and effective communication, care of the dying patient requires a specific

approach to clinical management. Care of the dying is urgent and needs to be focused, individually tailored, comprehensive and compassionate: all in the context of a limited time frame, when sub-standard care can have a disastrous impact on both patient and relatives for whom any adverse effects can live on through grief long after the patient has died. As Esther Rantzen describes:

> There are no rules. All deaths are different. Every patient has individual needs. If we get them wrong, or let them down, that failure will become a source of regret and sorrow. It can become a barrier that obscures all the happiest memories. That is why a good death is so important, if we can possibly achieve it. It is the key to remembering a good life. (2006: 7)

Providing care for the dying can at times be complex and challenging, especially for those less experienced in end of life care. However, when a good death is achieved, it can be a rewarding, satisfying experience for healthcare staff, knowing that they have provided the best possible care to patient and relative at the time of greatest need. The Liverpool Care Pathway for the dying patient (LCP) aims to promote good care in the last hours and days of life by helping less experienced healthcare staff provide optimum care for both patient and family.

KEY POINTS

- Good care of dying patients is an important skill for all healthcare professionals.
- The LCP is designed to facilitate good care for dying patients in the last hours/days of life.
- The LCP supports clinical decision-making to promote symptom control, comfort care, psychological and spiritual support for patients and their families in the last hours/days of life.

DISCUSSION

Background of the LCP

The LCP was developed to translate the best practice of caring for dying patients seen in hospices, where a relatively small percentage of the population die, to the hospital setting where the majority of population deaths occur (Office of National Statistics, 2005: 56). The emergence of hospital-based specialist palliative care teams has assisted with the incorporation of palliative care practice into the acute hospital sector. However, it remains that the majority of hospital-based dying patients are cared for by non-palliative care specialists, who may have limited end of life care experience (Kinder and Ellershaw, 2003: 11). The LCP is an integrated care pathway which can be used by healthcare professionals from all backgrounds, to help provide good quality care for dying patients. In addition to being a template for care of the dying within clinical practice, the LCP also has significance as an educational tool for staff training and development. There are three main sections to the LCP: initial assessment, ongoing care and care after death. Each section is further divided into a number of goals. Before commencing these sections, it is first necessary to decide whether the LCP is indicated.

Initiating the LCP

The LCP has been designed with a specific focus of providing care in the last hours/days of life for those whose death is expected. It is not intended for use in sudden unexpected death situations. Therefore the key step when initiating the LCP is that the multi-professional team managing the patient agrees that he or she is dying, that is expected to die within the next few days. Coming to this decision can be a complex and challenging process, influenced by a number of variables. Experienced healthcare professionals consider a variety of factors when coming to this decision (Stevenson and Ellershaw 2008: 411). This includes consideration of the patient's underlying medical diagnosis, the deterioration of this medical condition concurrent with a progressive worsening of physical, mental and functional ability. It is also important to consider any potentially reversible causes for the patient's deteriorating condition, where appropriate treatment may help improve general functioning and symptom control. It is a prerequisite for initiating the LCP that these potentially reversible causes have been considered. The exact pattern of signs and symptoms indicating the dying phase will be different for each individual patient. There may also be occasions when patients felt to be in the dying phase improve and stabilise for a period of time. These issues indicate why recognising the last days of life, or 'diagnosing dying' can be challenging. This reinforces the importance of taking a multi-professional approach, drawing on the different skills and experiences contributed by each discipline, with regular review of the patient's individual circumstances.

Section 1: Initial assessment

This first phase of initial assessment covers the key goals to be considered when the patient has entered the last hours/days of life. It begins by a baseline assessment of symptom control, establishing what the current problems are so care can be planned accordingly. This is followed by a series of goals covering the commonly occurring issues to be considered. The first goals relate to comfort measures concerning the adaptation of the clinical management plan to provide appropriate symptom control focused care. Current medication is assessed and reviewed and any that are non-essential discontinued. Oral drugs that are to be continued are converted to the subcutaneous route, potentially delivered via a continuous subcutaneous infusion if appropriate. As required (PRN) medication for the five key symptoms that may occur in the last hours/days of life should be prescribed. The LCP contains guidance for symptom control of pain, nausea and vomiting, agitation, respiratory tract secretions and breathlessness. A review of the interventional aspects of the care plan is prompted, with a focus on maintaining symptom control and comfort. Subsequent initial assessment goals focus on assessing and providing psychological and spiritual support for both patient and family, including their insight into the recognition of dying. This links to the final initial assessment goals dealing with communication issues, with the patient where possible, the family and wider healthcare team.

Section 2: Ongoing care

Section two continues the focus on maximising patient comfort through ongoing review of the symptom control, psychological and spiritual goals described in the initial assessment. For the duration that the patient remains on the LCP, assessment of these goals is performed on a four-hourly basis for inpatient units or at each visit in the community. The LCP acts as a template for multi-disciplinary documentation of care during the last hours/days of life. This includes documentation of care goal achievement, or if not achieved, a variance is recorded and subsequent action also documented. Monitoring of any continuous subcutaneous infusions used for medication delivery is included in the ongoing assessment phase.

Section 3: Care after death

This section concerns the death of the patient and subsequent procedures. Details of the death are recorded, including time/date and any persons present at time of death. These details aid completion of the required official death certification procedures. This section also focuses on ensuring appropriate procedures for the care of the body and any belongings after death. This includes any specific religious requirements that may be necessary. As in the previous sections, support of family/carers, who are now recently bereaved, is an important aspect of the LCP. It ensures that the family receives both practical information about registering the death and funeral arrangements, but also continuing psychological support and bereavement advice.

LCP development

From its beginnings in Liverpool, the LCP has spread both nationally in the UK and internationally, used in a range of healthcare settings (MCPCIL, 2008). It is part of national recommended policy, having been highlighted as a quality marker in the End of Life Care Strategy (Department of Health, 2009: 15). The LCP continues to be refined and developed through the work of the Marie Curie Palliative Care Institute, University of Liverpool, such as the National Care of the Dying Audit process (MCPCIL/RCP: 2007). Documents supporting the LCP have been developed, including relative information leaflets, specialised medication guidance for renal failure and LCP versions catering for specific circumstances such as Intensive Care Units. The LCP continues in its aim to raise the quality of care of the dying to the best possible standard for all. As Professor Mike Richards describes: 'How we care for the dying must surely be an indicator of how we care for all our sick and vulnerable patients. Care of the dying is urgent care; with only one opportunity to get it right to create a potential lasting memory for relatives and carers' (2007: 1).

PRACTICAL APPLICATION OF THE CONCEPT

Mrs X has a history of breast cancer with lung metastases. During an admission to hospital, her condition deteriorates, she becomes drowsy and unable to manage oral medication. Blood tests reveal no evidence of a potentially reversible cause for her deterioration. On discussion among the multi-professional team it is felt she is dying and the LCP is commenced.

Her regular medication is rationalised and PRN subcutaneous medications for symptom control are prescribed according to the guidance on the LCP. Her spiritual needs are assessed and it is arranged for her to be seen by a priest. The plan of care, including use of the LCP, is discussed with her family.

Her needs are monitored every four hours and the care plan is adjusted where needed. She dies peacefully two days later. Her family feel well supported by the clinical team. After her death, they are given information about registering the death and funeral arrangements in addition to information about bereavement services if required.

See also: *death; multi-disciplinary team; symptom management: common symptoms*

FURTHER READING

Clinical Guidelines Working Party, National Council for Palliative Care (NCPC), (1997, Reviewed and Updated November 2006) *Changing Gear: Guidelines for Managing the Last Days of Life in Adults.* London: National Council for Palliative Care (NCPC).

Ellershaw, J.E. and Wilkinson, S. (eds) (2003) *Care of the Dying: A Pathway to Excellence.* Oxford: Oxford University Press.

Ellershaw, J.E. and Ward, C. (2003) 'Care of the dying patient: the last hours or days of life'. *British Medical Journal*, 326: 30–4.

REFERENCES

Department of Health (2009) *End of Life Care Strategy – Quality Markers and Measures for End of Life Care.* Available at: www.dh.gov.uk/en/Publicationsandstatistics/Publications/PublicationsPolicyAndGuidance/DH_101681, accessed 13 July 2009.

Kinder, C. and Ellershaw, J.E. (2003) 'How to use the Liverpool Integrated Care Pathway for the dying patient?', in J.E. Ellershaw and S. Wilkinson (eds), *Care of the Dying: A Pathway to Excellence.* Oxford: Oxford University Press, pp. 11–41.

Marie Curie Palliative Care Institute Liverpool (MCPCIL)/Royal College of Physicians (RCP) Clinical Effectiveness & Evaluations Unit (CEEu) (2007) *National Care of the Dying Audit – Hospitals(NCDAH) Generic Report 2006/2007.* Available at: www.rcplondon.ac.uk/college/ceeu/NCDAH/NCDAH-Generic-Report.pdf, accessed 27 June 2009.

symptom management: LCP

217

Marie Curie Palliative Care Institute Liverpool (MCPCIL) (2008) *What is the LCP? – Healthcare professionals*, available at: www.liv.ac.uk/mcpcil/liverpool-care-pathway/index.htm, accessed 29 June 2009.

Office of National Statistics (ONS) (2005) 'Mortality statistics – series 38', available at: www.statistics.gov.uk/downloads/theme_health/Dh1_38_2005/DH1_No_38.pdf, accessed 29 June 2009.

Rantzen, E. (2006) 'Foreword', in J. Feinmann, C. Peterson, D.R. Goldhill, J.E. Ellershaw, S. Noble and D. Beckerman (eds), *How to Have a Good Death*. London: Dorling Kindersley Publishers Ltd.

Richards, M. (2007), in Marie Curie Palliative Care Institute Liverpool (MCPCIL)/Royal College of Physicians (RCP) Clinical Effectiveness & Evaluations Unit (CEEu) (2007) 'National Care of the Dying Audit – Hospitals (NCDAH) Generic Report 2006/2007', Available at: www.rcplondon.ac.uk/college/ceeu/NCDAH/NCDAH-Generic-Report.pdf, accessed 27 June 2009.

Stevenson, J. and Ellershaw, J.E. (2008) 'Prognostication in the imminently dying patient', in P. Glare and N. Christakis (eds), *Prognosis in Advanced Cancer*. Oxford: Oxford University Press.

47 spirituality

The Reverend Ian Delinger

DEFINITION

For the patient and their loved ones, coming to terms with end of life can raise issues involving spirituality. This can be accompanied by a mature and well-formed faith, an emergence of a latent faith or no faith, which can lead to questions, distress and anxiety. Care from the perspective of spirituality issues must be acknowledged by healthcare professionals, who can be key figures in the exploration of faith and spirituality at the bedside, with the assistance of chaplains and faith leaders, because of the time they will spend and the trust they build with a patient, in which profound interactions occur.

KEY POINTS

This chapter will explore:

- the issues that arise as one approaches death, with particular focus on the Western Christian perspective;

- making sense of the faith and spirituality issues that might be expressed by the patient and their loved ones;
- approaches for healthcare professionals to help with meeting those spiritual needs and concerns.

DISCUSSION

With the clear understanding that the time of death is important, meaningful and often stressful for people of all faiths and none, this chapter mainly focuses on the spiritual needs of those who are of or, mostly, influenced by Western Christianity. Of all the religions, Western Christianity has most influenced British culture, and has a very developed practice of pastoral care to those who are dying. By and large, the other major faiths within Britain have very specific beliefs and practices regarding death and burial, but less of a focus on the care of those who are dying, as indicated by Orchard (2001: 153).

Unfortunately, the Church has become increasingly knowledge-focused, with less emphasis on experiencing God. As a result, those who have little experience of worship may find that their end of life issues that have a spiritual dimension are meaningless because of a lack of religious knowledge. What might be 'spiritual language' is expressed as 'psychological language', when in reality what one might be *experiencing* is an 'ineffable spirituality' because there is no language to express these experiences. However, given the opportunity, one can explore and experience, and seek the 'other' through which hopelessness and meaninglessness are lessened.

Issues that arise

At the time of death, some of the issues that may arise with either or both the patient and the loved ones include:

- Why – If there is a God, why does God allow me to suffer? What about the suffering of my loved ones? Will they cope without me?
- Who – Who am I as a person, and what has been accomplished or unfinished in life that may affect who I might be in any sort of afterlife?
- What – What happens when I die? At the moment of death? What is 'eternal life' and will I have it?
- Where – Where am I going after I die? Where/What/Who is 'on the other side'? Is there a Heaven and a Hell?
- How – How will I be judged once I am gone? What will people say at my funeral? If there is a God, how will 'I meet my Maker'? Am I worthy of an afterlife, or of the love of those left behind?

Making sense

Modern practice is informed by theology. The Death of Jesus includes the care and concern of the person, and incorporates Jesus's divinity and His Death's impact on Humanity. For many Christians, as described by the Doctrine Commission of the Church of England (DCCE), the commemoration of Jesus's Resurrection and anticipation of His Second Coming both at Easter or when there is Communion, emphasises a notion of an afterlife, which involves judgment and *eternal* life (Doctrine Commission, 1995: 193). These events are significant because they inform the British cultural understanding of life and death, however rightly or wrongly. Borne of Britain's Christian history is the concept of Heaven and Hell, and even those who do not believe in them may carry it within their subconscious. But, as the DCCE reports, fewer people believe, or contemplate, that humans are both body and soul (1995: xii), so at the point of death, the critical question arises: 'What next?'

Misconceptions about Christianity are alongside the portrayal of a rule-based religion, particularly when those rules are broken. From this, the 'Why, Who, What, Where and How' of dying can emerge for both the patient and loved ones: 'Do my beliefs fit into the rules?' which can colour the spiritual dimension in a palliative care setting. But it needs to be 'demystified' for patients and loved ones, *as well as* healthcare professionals. It is key to move from understanding taking precedence, and move toward the *experience* of a Merciful God who came to die for Humanity, and who took the 'sting' out of death (*The Bible*: 1 Corinthians 15.55).

Approaches

Practical, common-sense approaches to caring for the spiritual dimensions of patients and loved ones are best. Consider the person: the person of the patient *and* of the healthcare professional.

To be understanding, open to their vulnerability, and in touch with your own vulnerability is helpful. Being uncomfortable around or avoiding a patient's expressions of religious or spiritual concepts may cause more anxiety. A nurse does not have to have all the answers, although within the constraints of other duties, listening with genuine attentiveness may be all that is required. As indicated by Chapman, it may be easier to talk to someone who is not a close friend or member of the family (1995: 12).

Understanding the factual basics of the practices of various religions is helpful. Though, spiritual care requires only two things:

- First, be open to them as human beings. Every patient is more than just their ailment. Be open to explore the 'other' or the metaphysical.
- Second, understand your own spirituality, what you do and do not believe, in order to be open to discussing various beliefs and concepts.

Nurses are pulled onto the spiritual journeys of patients and loved ones. Finding the right metaphysical location to be in on that journey, without being drawn in too deeply or being too distant, requires patience, practice, and openness. Draw upon the Asklepian model of care, as described by Randall and Downie, which:

stresses the attention we must give to each patient with his or her story. There is no science or social science which can substitute for this. Palliative care professionals must not hide their human gaze behind questionnaires, counselling, or quality of life scales. 'Tools' may mend the car but not the broken spirit!

… Palliative care is, and ought to remain, different from other specialities by retaining the Asklepian ideal of healing through focusing on the patient before us. (2006: 203)

Further exploration of the Asklepian model of care, with an eye toward its relevance to spirituality, is recommended.

Experienced colleagues, chaplains and faith leaders are there to help or take over when the situation is beyond one's capabilities. Care works best when carers work together. Additionally, if situations arise which lead to a level of spiritual depth never before encountered, supervision should be sought in order to engage with the experience and grow in maturity and confidence.

Nurses should be confident in allowing the spiritual aspect of themselves and of others to be *experienced* and to be *mysterious*: God, or the 'other', is present, and can be experienced, but we know not how.

If nurses are aware of the spiritual needs and journeys of those who are dying, and their loved ones, and are able to respond and provide care accordingly, the experience can be very positive. Death and the body are a brief part of what can be a much longer life experience. Spiritual experiences happen in the remaining time a patient is living, whether a week or a decade. The broader the experiences of healthcare professionals and the more open to spiritual needs, the more holistic the care is to persons who are a part of the *humanity* into which God came to experience the same pain, suffering and death which we all do.

PRACTICAL APPLICATION OF THE CONCEPT

The example chosen is one that is more common, subtle and can sometimes be missed. The extreme cases, in which a patient or family members go from strong faith to rejection of faith, or vice versa, are less common, and require a longer discussion than is feasible here.

Henry's wife passed away, and in the initial funeral visit, Henry revealed much of his childhood in which his parents were quite severe in their treatment of their children, with particular emphasis on their faith. Henry was deemed to be 'bad', and therefore was never baptised, but taken to church. In adulthood, Henry rejected all notions of faith, and over his life read about various secular philosophies in attempts to disprove to himself all notions of faith.

After several discussions about faith and non-faith, particularly about good, evil and the afterlife, Henry asked to attend church. He attended, mostly with curiosity and difficulty. Over a year, he sought more knowledge, but also continued to experience through worship. Henry, on his own initiative, requested to be baptised. After preparation, Henry in his mid-seventies was baptised and confirmed by the bishop, along with other candidates much younger than he.

These thoughts undoubtedly began before Henry's wife died, and are not limited to those with previous Christian upbringings. Nurses who observe the subtle signs while the family and patient are in the hospital can be very useful in helping them begin to express what seems inexpressible, by finding ways to 'give permission' to express spiritual thoughts. Also helpful is to offer to find the Chaplain, suggest that a minister come, or even that they spend some quiet time in the hospital Chapel.

See also: good death; holism

FURTHER READING

The Archbishops' Council (ed.) (2000) *A Time to Heal: A Contribution Towards the Ministry of Healing.* London: Church House Publishing.

Houldin, A.D. (2000) *Patients with Cancer.* Philadelphia, PA : Lippincott Williams & Wilkins.

Charlton, R. (ed.) (2005) *Primary Palliative Care: Dying, Death and Bereavement in the Community.* Abingdon: Radcliffe Medical Press.

Kuebler, K.K. et al., (2005) *Palliative Practices: An Inter-disciplinary Approach.* St Louis, MO: Elsevier Mosby.

REFERENCES

Chapman, C. (1995) *In Love Abiding: Responding to the Dying and Bereaved.* London: Triangle SPCK.

Doctrine Commission of the Church of England (1995) *The Mystery of Salvation.* Harrisburg, PA: Morehouse Publishing.

Orchard, H. (ed.) (2001) *Spirituality in Health Care Contexts.* London: Jessica Kingsley.

Randall, F. and Downie, S.R. (2006) *The Philosophy of Palliative Care.* Oxford: Oxford University Press.

48 stress and palliative care

Jan Woodhouse

DEFINITION

In this chapter the focus is on occupational stress in the palliative care setting. It is a topic that is well-researched, mainly by the nursing profession, but there are issues that affect all levels of healthcare workers who provide palliative care. The chapter starts with a definition of occupational stress and moves on to look at the concept of coping. From there sources of stress are identified, along with general and specific symptoms found in palliative care, before concluding with some specific strategies in order to alleviate occupational stress.

Occupational stress in palliative care, which may present as a disturbance of the metabolic balance or homeostasis causing physical or emotional outcomes, has been described as the state when the demands of the work environment exceed the employee's coping resources (Fillion et al., 2007; Lambert and Lambert, 2008; Nyatanga, 2009). The demands of the work environment, in the palliative care setting, are numerous and may appear limitless, whereas the coping resources of the individual are finite and dependent, as Maslow (1954) notes, on personality traits.

KEY POINTS

- Maslow's exploration of coping versus expression is useful.
- Sources of occupational stress in palliative care are identified.
- The consequences of stress produce a range of symptoms.
- Palliative care staff may require specific stress-relieving strategies.

DISCUSSION

Coping

To understand what is meant by coping it is useful to read the words of Maunder (2006: 29), who states:

when nurses put on their uniform, they often put on a performance of behaviour expected of them in their role and do not display emotions in the same way as they would outside work.

Here it can be seen that nurses, and other health professionals, who may or may not wear a uniform, suppress their normal means of expression when they step into role, where coping is the expected behaviour. As far back as 1954, Maslow identified the differences between coping versus expression. Coping, he suggested, requires effort; can be learned; is a conscious act; has a purpose; requires motivation and can be determined by the environment and culture. Expression, on the other hand, is effortless; is released or disinhibited; is unconscious; is uncontrolled; and is personal rather than dictated by the environment or culture. Because coping requires effort it can be regarded as emotional work (Maunder, 2006). One factor that helps to support individuals in their emotional work (or labour) is the sense of community provided by colleagues, so it is a positive note that personnel working in palliative care often feel more supported than other healthcare settings (Aranda, 2004).

SOURCES OF STRESS AFFECTING HEALTHCARE GROUPS

Fillion et al. (2007) suggest that sources affecting stress can be split into three areas – professional, emotional and organisational.

Professional

Doctors, for example, dislike the sense of failure they experience when faced with a patient who has palliative care needs (Hanratty et al., 2006). They may struggle to find the right words, and may consider the patient 'a burden with no return' (2006: 495). They have limited time to spend with the patients and relatives, and have difficulties in prognostics. Some of the medical profession may see palliative care as something nurses do, because they have the necessary skill, and perceive that nurses have more time to spend with the patient and relatives.

However, the time factor may be illusionary, for nurses also report that they have a lack of time to spend with those in their care (Fillion et al., 2007; Holst et al., 2009). It is often nurses who have a detailed knowledge of the patient and their family, which may have a dysfunctional dynamic, and can further impact on the stress experienced (Holst et al., 2009). Nurses are also the predominate group that witness repeated episodes of pain and suffering in their constant caring for individuals with life-limiting illnesses, and the distress that accompanies death (Nyatanga, 2009). However, other groups such as physiotherapists, domestic and clerical staff, religious leaders and social workers may also be witness to such events and are often over-looked in stress-relieving strategies.

Emotional

The emotional aspect of the roles of healthcare workers are not totally suppressed as perhaps Maslow's 'coping versus expression' model seems to suggest. Instead healthcare workers utilise the positive elements of expression, rather than negative ones. Staff may feel intense emotional involvement and that the culture of niceness can contribute to feelings of stress (Nyatanga, 2009). Aranda (2004: 624) states that 'being nice or good is a central value in palliative care' but it comes at a cost. We sometimes have to recognise that we cannot be nice and good all of the time. Hence we may need channels where we can work out the negative emotions that get suppressed.

During the care of the patients staff are often exposed to existential questioning (Sabo, 2008) and moral dilemmas and distress (Pendry, 2007). This may cause individuals to call into question their own values and standards – wondering what they might do in the same circumstance of the patient or their relatives, wondering if their own belief system is strong enough to support them if faced with a similar situation, wondering who they are and what their purpose is in life. If there is no time to reflect on these important questions, the individual may feel emotionally over-loaded.

Organisational

Within the organisation several factors may causes stress. Most commonly cited are lack of resources, increasing workload, tensions between disciplines and their professional belief systems, lack of staff, role conflict, lack of time to relax or grieve, high levels of change, poor interpersonal relationships and diminishing job satisfaction (Aranda, 2004; Fillion et al., 2007; Nyatanga, 2009). Often it may be the line manager who is vilified for being the cause of the stress, when the reality is that there is a combination of factors that are well out of the control of the manager.

Today organisations are far more aware of the consequences of stress and make strenuous attempts in monitoring staff sickness and absenteeism, in order to identify where problems are arising.

Consequences of stress

There are a plethora of cognitive, physical, emotional and behavioural symptoms that may indicate an individual is suffering the effects of general stress (Lambert and Lambert, 2008). These symptoms have been collated into Table 48.1. Lambert and Lambert (2008) highlight that the symptoms may not always be due to stress, but can be part of another underlying physical or psychological condition.

Nyatanga (2009) notes that stress can be contagious and therefore you may find several people within a team who are experiencing symptoms at the same time. He also comments that stress has been identified as a factor in speeding up the ageing process.

Table 48.1 Symptoms of stress

Cognitive	Physical	Emotional	Behavioural
Memory impairment	Headaches	Moodiness	Eating more, or less
Indecisiveness	Backache	Agitation	Sleeping more, or less
Inability to	Muscle tension	Restlessness	Isolating oneself from
concentrate	Gastric	Short temper	others
Poor judgement	disturbances	Irritability	Procrastinating
Difficulty to think	Nausea	Impatience	Neglecting
clearly	Dizziness	Unable to relax	responsibilities
Thinking negatively	Sleep disturbances	Feeling tense	Using substances
Anxiety	Chest pain	Feeling	(alcohol, drugs or
Worrying	Raised pulse rate	overwhelmed	cigarettes) to relax
Loss of objectivity	Weight change	Feeling lonely	Nail biting
Fearfulness	Skin problems	or isolated	Pacing
	Reduced libido	Depression	Teeth grinding
	Frequent colds or		Jaw clenching
	infections		Overdoing activities
			Overreacting to
			unexpected problems
			Picking fights with
			others

Source: Lambert and Lambert (2008: 39)

There are other aspects that may be particular to the palliative care setting and are worth recording.

- Vicarious traumatisation (Sabo, 2008).
- Compassion fatigue (Aranda, 2004; Sabo, 2008; Holst et al., 2009).
- Distancing (Blomberg and Sahlberg-Blom, 2007; Maunders, 2006).
- Burnout (Aranda, 2004; Sabo, 2008).

Individuals may recognise that their coping mechanisms are exhausted and consequently they may possibly resign from the job (Pendry, 2007), resulting in a lost opportunity to support them and lost expertise.

Strategies to deal with occupational stress in palliative care

Lambert and Lambert (2008) repeat some well-known stress-busting strategies: avoid unnecessary stress, alter the situation, accept the things you cannot change, adapt to the stressor and take care of personal needs. While these mantras are useful for general stress, it is probably the latter two, those of adaptation and taking care of oneself, that are probably more useful in the reality that is palliative care, as the first three are part of the healthcare worker's role.

A naturally occurring phenomenon is 'dark' humour (Maunder, 2006), which may be a protective mechanism against emotional labour. Similarly there emerges a public emotion system, which differs from the private emotion system. Healthcare professionals who are 'on show' for the whole of their shift may not have the opportunity to utilise their private emotion system, so a strategy to overcome this is to ensure that staff take breaks away from the public's gaze.

Holst et al. (2009) discuss how the tension caused by dysfunctional families can be offset by using a seven-point plan. The plan involves maintaining a focus on palliative principles; maintaining flexibility; maintaining neutrality, transparency and professionalism; avoiding 'splitting' or divisions between staff; avoiding demonising; setting necessary limits; and having an intervention that involves multidisciplinary discussion, counselling and debriefing.

These latter two aspects would come into the notion of 'endings', a term used in counselling where relationships are described as having beginnings, middles and endings. So a stress-relieving strategy may be to formalise the idea of an ending by either having clinical supervision, or sending a card to relatives, attending the funeral or a memorial service, having informal conversations with colleagues, or expressing it through an artistic form, for example, writing poetry, stories, reflections, and producing art work.

PRACTICAL APPLICATION OF THE CONCEPT

While working as a ward manager Sarah had witnessed many deaths over the years. The ward she managed was very busy and an outbreak of winter vomiting virus had recently increased the demand on the beds as well as reducing the number of healthy staff. At the same time Sarah been had involved in the care of a person who was near to Sarah's age. Sarah had got to know the family well and had taken a pride in being the link between the medical management of the patient and being the one to explain issues to the patient and the family. The death of the patient, when it came, was very sudden due to a carotid haemorrhage and Sarah had spent a frantic time trying to control the bleeding, before administering sedation until the patient died. She then had to track down the family, who had gone shopping for food, and explain what had happened. Within half an hour of the patient's body being taken to the mortuary, a new patient was admitted to the now empty bed. Several days later Sarah found her thoughts returning to the scene that she had witnessed and she felt unable to do the things that she had planned for her much-needed day off. On returning to work, her colleagues noticed that she was acting irritably, and spending more and more time in the office or away from the ward.

See also: *caring for carers; multi-disciplinary teams*

FURTHER READING

Katz, R.S. and Johnson, T.A. (eds) (2006) *When Professionals Weep: Emotional and Counter-transference Responses in End-of-life Care*. Abingdon: Routledge.

Payne, S., Seymour, J. and Ingleton, C. (eds) (2004) *Palliative Care Nursing: Principles and Evidence for Practice*. Maidenhead: Open University Press.

Speck, P. (2006) *Teamwork in Palliative Care*. Oxford: Oxford University Press.

REFERENCES

Aranda, S. (2004) 'The cost of caring: surviving the culture of niceness, occupational stress and coping strategies', in S. Payne, J. Seymour and C. Ingleton (eds), *Palliative Care Nursing: Principles and Evidence for Practice*. Maidenhead: Open University Press, pp. 620–35.

Blomberg, K. and Sahlberg-Blom, E. (2007) 'Closeness and distance: a way of handling difficult situations in daily care', *Journal of Clinical Nursing*, 16: 244–54.

Fillion, L., Tremblay, I., Truchon, M., Côté, D., Struthers, C.W. and Dupuis, R. (2007) 'Job satisfaction and emotional distress among nurses providing palliative care: empirical evidence for an integrative occupational stress model', *International Journal of Stress Management*, 14(1): 1–25.

Hanratty, B., Hibbert, D., Mair, F., May, C., Ward, C., Corcoran, G., Capewell, S. and Litva, A. (2006) 'Doctor's understanding of palliative care', *Palliative Medicine*, 20: 493–7.

Holst, L., Lundgren, M., Olsen, L. and Ishøy, T. (2009) 'Dire deadlines: coping with dysfunctional family dynamics in an end-of-life care setting', *International Journal of Palliative Nursing*, 15(1): 34–41.

Lambert, V.A. and Lambert, C.E. (2008) 'Nurses' workplace stressors and coping strategies', *Indian Journal of Palliative Care*, 14(1): 38–4.

Maslow, A.H. (1954) *Motivation and Personality*. New York: Harper & Row.

Maunder, E.Z. (2006) 'Emotion work in the palliative nursing care of children and young people', *International Journal of Palliative Nursing*, 12(1): 27–33.

Nyatanga, B. (2009) 'Are your shoelaces shortening?' *International Journal of Palliative Nursing*, 15(2): 55.

Pendry, P.S. (2007) 'Moral distress: recognising it to retain nurses', *Nursing Economics*, 25(4): 217–21.

Sabo, B.M. (2008) 'Adverse psychological consequences: compassion fatigue, burnout and vicarious traumatisation: are nurses who provide palliative and hematological [*sic*] cancer care vulnerable?', *Indian Journal of Palliative Care*, 14(1): 23–9.

49 technology: equipment procurement

Sonya Currey, Janice Foster and Virginia C. Williams

DEFINITION

The focus of this chapter is the procurement of community equipment in support of patients with life-limiting illness; discussing the effects of changes to community equipment procurement which are currently being piloted. *Transforming Community Equipment* (Department of Health, 2006) indicates its 'overriding principle as being that improvements or changes must centre on the interests of the individual'. Recognition of the need for a timely, individualised response to equipment needs in support of independent living is evident in its rhetoric but there is scant reference to the needs of those nearing or receiving end of life care.

Can the current focus of these proposed changes allow sufficient flexibility to respond to the often acutely arising needs experienced by those patients at end of life? Provision of resource in the form of equipment to support 'needs-based' care within the patient's home is an essential ingredient of the care package required to respond to this patient group which by its very nature (unpredictable and declining health status) demands a sensitive yet efficient response. Due to the physical decline encountered during the terminal phase of disease, the equipment required is not only to optimise an individual's well-being and achievement of their Preferred Priorities of Care (PPC) but also to support carers and healthcare providers in safely meeting nursing need. This equipment more often than not includes large pieces such as profiling bed frames, lifting equipment, recliner chairs, mobile commodes and pressure-relieving equipment and therefore relies on a sufficiently robust delivery system.

KEY POINTS

The following points are considered to form the core components of the procurement process:

- background/history,
- availability of equipment,
- referral process,
- delivery of equipment,
- disposal of equipment.

DISCUSSION

Background/history

Recent triggers for reconsidering the concept of equipment provision include Audit Commission reports (2000, 2002), concurrent studies by the Department of Health (2006) and Winchcombe and Mandelstam (2006), all of which highlighted geographical disparity in the provision of community equipment. The political directive (Department of Health, 2006) sets out a non-mandatory framework for future equipment services, which is currently being piloted in three areas in the North West (Winchcombe and Mandelstam, 2008). This proposes increased choice with the potential to try out equipment (at Disable

Living Centres) for service users who have the time and ability to use the system, and for whom the equipment will aid independence.

The model sets out to create more routes to assessment, allowing referrals to be initiated by any health professional or by patients themselves. It then requires an independent assessment in support of individual equipment needs, the pool of assessors may require further development which will obviously take time for this to be achieved. In the interim, District Nurses (DN) fill the breach and are required to carry out this assessment to facilitate a prescription for equipment prior to the items being delivered to the patient's home. While the majority of items may be available within target times, Moran (2008) already highlights a need to review the storage and delivery strategy for equipment likely to be needed in support of end of life care (beds, hoists and pressure area care items). This extra burden on nursing time plus the delay in receiving equipment as a consequence of the additional assessment/ delivery delays are issues to be addressed urgently; consequently having the potential to impact upon the patient's PPC and subsequent quality of life.

Availability of equipment

Currently a dual process exists in the form of equipment on prescription, which is generated by an appropriately trained assessor and dispensed by an approved commercial retailer (the retail model) or through a centralised distribution centre (the integrated community equipment store model). However, Moran (2008) identifies a 23–26% year-on-year growth rate in demand for equipment, arising from the demographic challenges posed by an ageing population with subsequent and ongoing expansion of the equipment and supporting staff resource pool being imperative. The Department of Health (2006) suggests demand forecasting at a local level based on population data, joint health and social care requirements for equipment and actual spend is vital to ensure availability of such a resource pool. Suggestion that large retail outlets and supermarkets may possibly stock a wider variety of equipment have yet to materialise, however, this has the potential to reach a wider patient group and enhance patient choice inclusive of styles and colour. However, the aesthetic appeal has limited value for those at end of life.

Referral process

Procurement via the retail model, for those requiring long-term use of equipment, is initiated through the selection of the appropriate pathway. Those requiring long-term use will require assessment necessitating the negotiation of at least an eight-phase pathway with lengthy time implications rendering it unwieldy for those at end of life. Therefore, the short-term pathway has the potential to meet need through loans dependent on the flexibility of the supporting contract arrangements; this is again initiated by the same lengthy paperwork.

However, in comparison the Integrated Community Equipment Services (ICES) model is initiated by a user friendly tick list with supporting evidence to ensure prioritisation for those at end of life. Dependent on the geographical locality, further validation may be required for specific pieces of equipment (pressure-relieving) from tissue viability nurses.

Delivery of equipment

Equipment specific to end of life care requires delivery as opposed to collection and is dependent on logistical organisation for an optimised response. Moran (2008) is already suggesting that a two-tier system may be required to achieve the performance indicators of seven days for aids supporting independent living (delivered from regional suppliers) and to facilitate sameday equipment provision required for those at end of life. The maintenance of local satellite centres may be required to ensure the latter need is met; therefore questioning the effectiveness of disbanding the ICES model if the retail model pilots are deemed successful.

Disposal of equipment

The overriding principle is that any improvement or change must centre on the interests of the individual (Department of Health, 2006). How then can we support the notion of disposable rather than recyclable equipment? It may be that disposable items are the most economically viable option in the short term, avoiding the costs of collecting and decontaminating equipment for reuse. However, consideration of the long-term impact on the environment and subsequently on the individual for whom the equipment was first prescribed appears to have been overlooked.

Summary

The impetus for redeveloping the equipment procurement service arose from a number of triggers; most recently the Audit Commission reports (2000, 2002) and a coinciding Department of Health (2006) review of community equipment services. The resulting political directive sets out a currently non-mandatory framework for future equipment service development moving from the ICES to a retail model of provision. The latter system supports an increased choice for service users, which could be of benefit for those patients who have long-term illness, and who have a prognosis conducive to negotiating the lengthy procedure and target times for delivery. However, the authors' concerns lie in the revised services' ability to meet the needs of those patients with life limiting illness and resulting palliative care needs, who may find that time is too short to wait in line for the allocation and delivery of equipment. The facilitation of quality of life and PPC at end of life demands a more robust and responsive service to support the often unpredictable and rapidly changing needs of this vulnerable group in choosing where to spend their last days of life.

PRACTICAL APPLICATION OF THE CONCEPT

Harry, an independent widow with an active social life was admitted (post cord compression) to the hospice. During his admission he acknowledged his poor prognosis and identified his PPC as home. Harry had little support at his own home but suggested a compromise of his son's home in a neighbouring locality.

Harry experienced rapid disease progression, he recognised that he was dying and wanted to be discharged. Planning to facilitate Harry's PPC became paramount. A care package was agreed, equipment referral generated and a discharge date set for 24 hours later.

Despite the DNs being able to support this discharge, Harry's PPC being his son's address resulted in the equipment referral being dealt with by a community loans department which was piloting a new procurement system (Department of Health, 2006). This system required an independent equipment assessment by the DN to generate a prescription which then facilitated delivery of equipment, the process taking up to 72 hours. Consequently Harry's discharge was delayed to coincide with equipment delivery; this was time that Harry could ill afford.

Harry died in the hospice, unable to achieve his dying wish.

See also: death; environment of care; patient choice and preferences in palliative care

FURTHER READING

Dunne, K., Sullivan, K. and Kernoham, G. (2005) 'Palliative care for patients with cancer: district nurses experiences', *Journal of Advanced Nursing*, 50(4): 372–80.

Winchcombe, M. (2008) 'Making disability equipment ordinary: choice, control and the retail model', *International Journal of Therapy and Rehabilitation*, 15(3): 115–18.

Wright, K. (2002) 'Caring for the terminally ill: the District Nurses' perspective', *British Journal of Nursing*, 11: 18.

REFERENCES

Audit Commission (2000) *Fully Equipped: The Provision of Equipment to Older or Disabled People by the NHS and Social Services in England and Wales*. London: Audit Commission.

Audit Commission (2002) *Fully Equipped Update 2002: Assisting Independence*. London: Audit Commission.

Department of Health (2006) *Transforming Community Equipment Services and Wheelchair Programme* (TCEWS). London: DH.

Heap, S. (2008) *The Cheshire Community Equipment Services Update*. Community services, April 2008. London: Mark Allen Publishing Ltd

Moran, B. (2008) *Transforming Community Equipment: Transformation or Evolution?* Equipment services January 2008. London: Mark Allen Publishing Ltd

Winchcombe, M. and Mandelstam, M. (2006) *Getting on with our Lives*. Disabled Living North West, in partnership with Co-operative Bank.

Moyra A. Baldwin and Joanne Greenwood

DEFINITION

Value of Life is one of those concepts that is implied rather than explicitly explored in palliative care literature. Life, frequently, is valued only when it is under threat. This was depicted by Das in his 'Thought for the day' as he reflected on the Southern Australian bush-fires: 'Life can only be as good as our appreciation of it' (Das, 2009). Value of Life, and by implication its appreciation, are explored below. Value of Life is depicted as a model in Figure 50.1 as overlapping circles with the individual placed at the centre, demonstrating how individuals appraise life in order to find meaning and determine what Value of Life is for them.

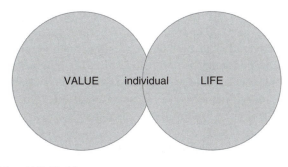

Figure 50.1   *Value of Life Model*

233

KEY POINTS

- Value of life is individual.
- Value of life is underpinned by each person's beliefs, attitude and experience.
- It is unique because individuals are personally affected from a biological, psychological and, ultimately, a sociological perspective. Thus it is dynamic.

DISCUSSION

When there is a threat to one's life or health it appears that it is at this time that the significance of value of life has meaning to the individual. This is also true for those around them: the family and friends who are affected by the individual's life changes. When there is an actual or perceived threat to one's life or health, value of life is, as Harris (1985: 16) claims, not a case of not knowing what it is but a case of there being 'so many answers'. By this we understand that there are many answers, or perceptions, about the meaning of value of life. Examples from everyday life, where re-evaluation of the meaning of value of life is considered, include life-changing events such as the threat of loss of life due to illness, or the experience of being given a diagnosis such as cancer or heart failure. Others include those where a significant portion of the population is involved, for example, the many lives lost in Australia that Das spoke of in his reflection, in 2009. The 'credit crunch' that is consuming a large part of the world at the end of the first decade of the twenty-first century has also brought about situations that are ripe for people to reflect on, and consider, the value of life for them. This was denoted by Anderson (2009) in a BBC interview, and his book *Cityboy* in which he realises that there is more to life than monetary gain. Value of life is demonstrated, to some degree, in the discussion and examples below.

Value of Life: pre-illness

The concept Value of Life can be said to lie within an individual's subconscious thoughts. It is at the point of a life-threatening diagnosis that thoughts become part of consciousness whereby feelings, thoughts and emotions are activated. This may trigger feelings such as anxiety, agitation, numbness and despondency as one realises that life may never be the same again. According to Harris (1985), what is considered as Value of Life is that which the individual perceives to be value of life, in other words, it is unique to each and every one of us, and is dynamic.

Value of Life – under threat

In the foreword to Rollason's autobiography Lynam (2000) praised Helen Rollason's courage when faced with a terminal cancer. He notes the example she gave to him, her child and others in the following words 'how we should hope to behave when we find ourselves under fire' (Lynam, in Rollason, 2000: ix). Illness gives one a changed perspective of Value of Life: changes as noted in a literature review conducted by Bassett (2002). Comparing nurses' perceptions of care and caring with those of patients' the author notes that perceptions, and here we infer Value of Life, are 'context dependent'. The person facing a terminal illness may be less interested about the physical aspects of care that might worry an acutely ill person, but be more concerned about issues with regard to what can be described as building, maintaining or

Table 50.1   Value of Life

V – Value/view of life
A – Attitude
L – Life
U – Unique
E – Experience

L – Losses
I – Individual
F – Future
E – Evaluate/re-evaluate

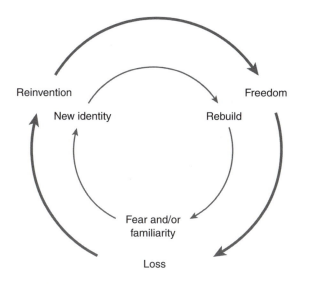

Figure 50.2   *Value of Life Spiral*

severing relationships. Thus there is a re-evaluation of what gives life meaning or purpose. This is depicted by the mnemonic Value of Life in Table 50.1.

Value of Life – at diagnosis

Diagnosis of a life-limiting illness involves the breaking of and receiving bad news (Faulkner, 1998; Buckman, 2001) which Buckman (1992: 2001) explains, for people who are hearing the bad news, is that news which affects their future. It requires one to adjust both to the present and revise future plans. Thus it involves revisiting one's concept of Value of Life. This is depicted in the Value of Life spiral (see Figure 50.2). The inner spiral represents the process of adjustment required and the outer spiral the potential outcome of such an adjustment. For the person who is informed that s/he has a cancer, or the person whose symptoms are confirmed as metastatic spread the diagnosis involves a changed perspective on life and the value of life. For some there will be a loss of hope, for others there will be hope, for example for relief of symptoms, or a peaceful death. The person's attitude to the diagnosis is influenced by and affects the value of life. In the event of diagnosis one's value of life can be critically threatened, however, in the event of a misdiagnosis it could be argued that hope is removed. On receiving the news that it is misdiagnosis hope may be replaced and value of life returned and reinvention may occur.

PRACTICAL APPLICATION OF THE CONCEPT

'Can one live with no kidney function and one lung?' John asked his family. John, a 49-year-old gentleman, had a long-standing diagnosis of chronic renal failure. Following investigations, that were not related to his renal failure, he was given a diagnosis of lung cancer: another life-limiting illness. This second diagnosis came at a time when John was adjusting to changes in his health, income and to the home haemo-dialysis treatment. John was valuing life as he lived with the condition, he viewed dialysis as a time of maintaining his condition and his life, a time between transplantation when life would start again. It was a period of transition, an interim measure, as he would say, 'I'll forget about this time once transplanted'. For John, life would start again, independence would be regained, as well as freedom. The challenge was that a new diagnosis had to make him rethink and re-evaluate the value of his life. John perceived he had Value of Life as he wanted to continue living, hence the question whether it was possible to survive with his multiple conditions. No matter what, John wanted to live.

Using the Value of Life Model (Figure 50.1) and mnemonic (Table 50.1) it can be seen that John was reflecting in both 'value' and 'life' areas and these confirmed, for John, that his life had value. For John the Value of life and his Attitude towards Life was an Unique Experience, while experiencing Losses that were Individual to him, that were physiological, psychological, and financial, he judged life in a positive manner, could envisage a Future and Evaluated outcomes in terms of value of (his) life.

Mary is 53-years-old with metastatic uterine cancer. She has been told that her breathing problems are due to secondaries and that she could be given chemotherapy for relief of symptoms. Mary is fully aware of her diagnosis and knows that without chemotherapy she is likely to die within weeks rather than months. Having experienced the side-effects of chemotherapy for the first cancer, for Mary the Value of Life and her Attitude towards Life was, again, a Unique Experience. While experiencing Losses that were Individual to her, that were physiological and psychological, one could say that she also judged life in a positive manner. Nevertheless, the Future she envisaged and the Evaluative outcomes could not outweigh the other less positive effects of treatment and progression.

Value of Life is dynamic: it varies in respect of context. In the examples of John and Mary, first impressions might suggest that John has a positive outlook on life as compared with Mary. This, of course, may be a matter of opinion. If we consider organ donation, families' perceptions may be that the individual is still alive within a different life, in another individual. It is one of the many reasons, perhaps, that families donate their loved ones organs. Additionally, it needs to be considered that the person who has received the organ also has a new meaning and value of life. The person may now feel free from some of the medical regimes that were previously restrictive. Therefore, it could be said there are some positive outcomes for both individuals, although one is not 'technically with us' on earth. Another example of the importance of context, and the creative and uniquely innovative aspects of Value of Life is Jade Goody, the TV reality star's much publicised palliative care journey. Jade's story raised awareness of cervical cancer and therefore valuing the life of others was a priority. It could also be argued that she was valuing the life of her young sons, prior to her untimely death, so that they had future financial security. Or, is the reality that it was probably a balance of somewhere in-between? It could be argued that even in death, individuals can contribute in some way to the value of life for themselves and others.

See also: loss, grief and bereavement; organ donation

FURTHER READING

Harris, J. (1985) *The Value of Life: An Introduction to Medical Ethics*. London: Routledge.

REFERENCES

Anderson, G. (2009) *'Cityboy': Beer and Loathing in the Square Mile*. London: Headline Book Publishing.
Bassett, C. (2002) 'Nurses' perceptions of care and caring', *International Journal of Nursing*, 8(1): 8–15.
Buckman, R. (1992) *How to Break Bad News*. London: Papermac.
Buckman, R. (2001) 'Communication in palliative care: a practical guide', in D. Dickenson, M. Johnson and J. S. Katz (eds), *Death, Dying and Bereavement*, 2nd edn. London: The Open University in association with Sage, pp.146–73.
Das, A. (2009) *Thought for the Day*. BBC Radio 4, 11 February 2009.
Faulkner, A. (1998) *When the News is Bad: A Guide for Health Professionals on Breaking Bad News*. Cheltenham: Stanley Thornes.
Harris, J. (1985) *The Value of Life: An Introduction to Medical Ethics*. London: Routledge.
Lynam, D. (2000) 'Foreword', in H. Rollason. *Life's Too Short: An Autobiography*. London: Hodder & Stoughton, pp. vii–ix.

value of life

index

Index

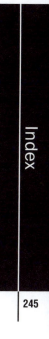

Index